Water for Survival

Essential Techniques, Tools, and Tips to Survive Any Water Emergency

Carlos Mack

Table of Contents

Introduction

Water is essential to life.

It is the most basic and fundamental human need.

We need water to survive, and yet, many of us take it for granted. We go about our daily lives without giving much thought to the water we consume. We turn on the faucet, and it's there. We flush the toilet, and it's gone. **But what if one day, water was not there?** What if we woke up to find that the taps were dry, and there was no water to be had?

It's a scenario that is difficult to imagine, but it's not as far-fetched as you might think. Droughts, floods, and natural disasters can all cause disruptions in the water supply. Wars and political upheavals can also have a significant impact on access to water. In short, water is not as abundant or as secure as we would like to believe. Even though our bodies are composed of up to 60% water, we still need to consume it every day to maintain good health. So what happens when access to clean water is compromised, such as in emergency situations? This is a question that has been posed to countless people, and the answer can often mean the difference between life and death.

Throughout history, water has played a crucial role in the development of civilizations. From ancient Mesopotamia to modern-day New York City, people have settled near bodies of water because of the vital role it plays in their daily lives. Rivers, lakes, and oceans provide food, transportation, and irrigation for crops. Water is a source of power, used for everything from grinding grain to generating electricity. The importance of water is evident in the names of many cities, such as Venice, Amsterdam, and Seattle, all of which are situated on waterways.

However, water can also be a source of danger. Floods, tsunamis, and hurricanes can all wreak havoc on communities that are unprepared for the deluge. Water can also be a carrier of disease, from cholera to typhoid fever. In fact, water-borne diseases are responsible for more deaths worldwide than any other cause.

The importance of water for survival cannot be overstated. It's something that we need to take seriously and prepare for. This is where my book comes in. Here's a brief summary of what you can expect to find in each chapter of the book. I will take a comprehensive look at the topic of water for survival situations. I will cover everything from the different types of water sources on our great planet, to the various methods of water purification available to you. Water storage options, proper sanitation of containers, and transportation of water in emergency situations will be covered. I will also look at how to prepare you, and your water supply, for natural disasters. I have researched different types of water-borne diseases, and will cover how they spread, and how to prevent them. Last, I will talk about the future and why it is so important to educate others on water conservation and help do our part to preserve this precious resource for generations to come.

Throughout the book, I will provide practical solutions and tips for individuals to prepare for emergencies as it relates to your #1 resource: **WATER!** To fully absorb and apply the information provided in this book, I recommend you take notes as you read. I know, I know, come on Carlos you are saying this sounds like school all over again!? It's just my suggestion, so no big deal if you decide note taking is not for you. However, I feel this will help all readers, no matter their skill level, on their journey. Taking notes can help to identify any knowledge gaps on topics that may require further research or study. These notes will then be written in your own words to be discovered in the future when called upon for reference. So, while reading this book, it is advisable to have a notebook or note-taking app on hand to jot down important points, new ideas, or questions that may arise. By doing so, readers will be able to engage more deeply with the material and apply the knowledge gained to their own unique situations for future projects or immediate purchases to improve their current situation. We are all at various stages of preparation so I just want to be clear on that point. Also, I understand the book can be read cover to cover of course, but may be best applied in your life as a look-up guide down the road.

These steps are critical for individuals to take to ensure their safety and well-being in a crisis, and they can make all the difference in the world when clean water is not readily available.

In conclusion, this book is a must-read for anyone who is concerned about water for survival situations. Whether you're an outdoor enthusiast, a prepper, or just someone who wants to be prepared for any eventuality, this book has something for you. You can help ensure that clean water is accessible to all, even in the most challenging of circumstances. This researched collection of information on water for survival was thoughtfully organized to help provide a comprehensive understanding of the challenges faced in emergency situations, and how we can better prepare for them.

In today's uncertain economic and political climate, it's more important than ever to be prepared in our own homes and communities. This book is a solution to that problem, providing practical advice and guidance on how to ensure access to clean water in any situation. So for whatever the future may bring, start preparing NOW and don't wait until it's too late! Are you ready to learn the essential water survival skills? Keep reading.

Chapter 1:

Water Needs For Humans

"Thousands have lived without love, not one without water." –W.H. Auden

Water is a vital nutrient for human health and well-being. It is crucial to understand our daily water requirements, the effects of dehydration, and how to calculate the water needs of our families. So let's dive right in!

Daily Water Requirements

The daily water requirement for an adult is dependent on various factors such as gender, age, body weight, physical activity, and climate. On average, men require more water than women, and pregnant or breastfeeding women require more water than non-pregnant women. People who engage in physical activities that make them sweat, such as athletes, construction workers, or outdoor enthusiasts, require more water than those who are less active.

The climate can also affect the body's water needs. In hot or humid weather, the body loses water more rapidly through sweat, requiring an increase in water intake. Additionally, individuals living at higher elevations may need more water to counteract the effects of dry air. In cold and dry weather, a person may not feel as thirsty, but they still need to drink enough water to prevent dehydration.

As we age, our body's ability to conserve water decreases, which means that older adults may need to drink more water to stay hydrated. This demographic's kidneys may not function as efficiently, making older adults more susceptible to dehydration. Additionally, children have a higher water requirement per pound of body weight than adults because their bodies are still developing and they have higher metabolic rates.

Certain health conditions may affect a person's daily water requirements. Consult with a healthcare provider to determine these specific water needs.

Here are a few examples of those health conditions:

Diabetes: People with diabetes have an increased risk of dehydration, as high blood sugar levels can cause the body to lose more fluids through urine. Additionally, people with diabetes may need to drink more water to prevent high blood sugar levels and other complications.

Kidney disease: People with kidney disease may need to limit their fluid intake to prevent fluid buildup in the body. However, the exact amount of fluid restriction can vary depending on the stage of kidney disease and other factors.

Cystic fibrosis: People with cystic fibrosis have a higher salt content in their sweat, which means they need to drink more fluids to prevent dehydration and maintain a healthy balance of electrolytes.

Gastrointestinal conditions: People with gastrointestinal conditions, such as diarrhea or vomiting, may lose more fluids and electrolytes than normal, which means they need to drink more water to prevent dehydration.

The National Academies of Sciences, Engineering, and Medicine provide daily water intake recommendations, which vary depending on age and gender.

For adult men, it is recommended to consume about 3.7 liters (125 ounces) of water daily, and for adult women, it is recommended to consume about 2.7 liters (91 ounces) of water daily.

Age Group	Average Ounces of Water per Day
Adult Men	125 - 150 oz
Adult Women	91 - 125 oz
Children	45 - 64 oz

Water consumption is a crucial component for maintaining optimal bodily functions. To maintain proper hydration levels, stick to these suggested amounts daily. Despite the importance of water consumption, many individuals fail to drink enough water, leading to dehydration. In the next section, we will delve deeper into the topic of dehydration, exploring its causes, symptoms, and potential health consequences.

Understanding Dehydration

Dehydration is a condition that occurs when the body loses more water than it takes in, resulting in an imbalance of electrolytes in the body. Electrolytes are minerals that are essential for various bodily functions, such as maintaining fluid balance, regulating the body's pH, and transmitting nerve impulses.

Dehydration can be caused by various factors, such as intense physical activity, exposure to hot or humid weather, or an illness that causes vomiting or diarrhea.

Common signs and symptoms of dehydration include:

Thirst: Thirst is one of the earliest signs of dehydration. As the body loses water, it sends a signal to the brain that it needs more fluid to function properly.

Dark urine: Dehydration can cause the urine to become more concentrated and appear darker in color.

Dry mouth and throat: As the body loses water, it can lead to dryness of the mouth and throat.

Fatigue: Dehydration can cause fatigue and weakness, as the body does not have enough fluid to carry out normal bodily functions.

Dizziness and lightheadedness: Dehydration can cause a drop in blood pressure, which can lead to dizziness and lightheadedness.

In severe cases, dehydration can lead to seizures, kidney failure, heat stroke, or even death. It is crucial to recognize these symptoms, here are several ways to slow or stop it in its tracks.

Here are some facts and statistics on dehydration in the US:

Dehydration is a common issue in the US. As mentioned earlier, the recommended daily water intake for adults is about 2.7-3.7 liters (91-125 ounces) for men and 2.2-2.7 liters (74-91 ounces) for women. Still, an estimated 75% of American adults are chronically dehydrated!

Dehydration can lead to a range of health problems, including headaches, fatigue, dizziness, dry skin, constipation, and kidney stones.

A 2018 study found that only 22% of American adults drink enough water on a daily basis, and that more than a third of Americans don't drink any water at all.

Athletes and people who engage in physical activity are at a higher risk of dehydration, as they lose water through sweat.

Children and older adults are also at a higher risk of dehydration, as their bodies may not be as efficient at regulating fluid levels.

Certain groups of people, such as those with diabetes, kidney disease, or who take certain medications, may be at a higher risk of dehydration.

Ways to Stop Dehydration:

The good news is that there are several ways to prevent dehydration and ensure that your body stays hydrated. Here are a few of the most effective strategies for optimum fluid intake for humans.

Drink more water: This is obvious, but the most effective way to stop dehydration is to drink more water! For mild cases of dehydration, drinking water or other fluids that contain electrolytes can help replenish the body's fluids and electrolytes. To spice up this rather boring suggestion, try switching up water bottles or cups that you use for water consumption. Personally, I will go through as many as 5 different containers for good ol' H20 in a day, here is a what that may look like: Tervis with handle & straw at home, stainless cup with stainless straw at the office, a can of flavored spritzer water at lunch, a plain water bottle in the car, another style of open-mouth water bottle for exercising, or in my backpack for on-the-go consumption. Get creative with your water bottles and feel free to mix it up with straws, wide mouth containers, add ice, even flavors (just be careful of the added sugar). Variety is the spice of life! I say this often, but am now putting it in a book... I drink more water than anyone I know. I think one of the reasons for my successful water intake has to do with my subtle container mix-up to help confuse my subconscious that this may be a treat (not just plain old water in that stainless steel cup). This tends to reduce some of my cravings for soda, juice or an energy drink during most of my day. There is likely a psychological meaning behind that, potentially the "Mandela Effect", where I forget my mug has water in it, not a crisp and refreshing Coca-Cola instead. I still love red wine or cold beer, don't get me wrong, but on a day-to-day hydration basis, try this variation trick and let me know if it works for you.

Avoid diuretics: Diuretics, such as caffeine and alcohol, can cause the body to lose more fluid and worsen dehydration. It is best to avoid diuretics when dehydrated. As mentioned above, I enjoy a nice chewy glass of red wine or a cold IPA as much as the next person. However, when enjoying a coffee or libation, you will almost always find me with a glass of water to go along with it. News flash, coffee and wine are not water people! Limit your consumption and drink water with them, that is my best advice here. When diuretics are used excessively or inappropriately, they can lead to dehydration and electrolyte imbalances, which can cause symptoms such as thirst, fatigue, muscle cramps, and dizziness. So by all means enjoy a libation or 2, but just keep the intake in check as it pertains to overall hydration.

Stay in a cool place: High temperatures and humidity can cause the body to lose more water. Staying in a cool place or air conditioning can help prevent further dehydration.

Eat water-rich foods: Foods with high water content, such as watermelon, cucumber, and strawberries, can help increase fluid intake. So replace that sausage with a salad at lunch today and thank me tomorrow.

Seek medical attention: In severe cases of dehydration, medical attention may be necessary. IV fluids may be required to rehydrate the body.

It is essential to recognize the signs of dehydration and take immediate action to rehydrate the body. Drinking water or other fluids that contain electrolytes, such as sports drinks or coconut water, can quickly help replenish the body's fluids and electrolytes. In severe cases of dehydration, medical attention may be necessary, such as intravenous (IV) fluids.

Calculating a Family's Water Needs (for an Emergency)

Calculating a family's water needs is critical to ensure that they each have enough water stored for an emergency. When preparing for an emergency, it is recommended to have at least a **72-hour supply of water per person, which equates to about one gallon of water per person per day**. However, it is essential to consider each family's unique water needs, such as physical activity levels, age, and climate.

To calculate your family's daily water needs, start by estimating the number of people in the household and multiplying it by the recommended daily water intake for their gender and age group. For example, if there are four people in the household, two adult men, one adult woman, and a child, the estimated daily water needs would be:

2 adult men x 3.7 liters = 7.4 liters (250 ounces)

1 adult woman x 2.7 liters = 2.7 liters (91 ounces)

1 child x 1.5 liters = 1.5 liters (51 ounces)

Total estimated daily water needs for the household: 11.6 liters (392 ounces).

It is essential to factor in any additional water needs for a family, such as pets or medical needs. Additionally, it is crucial to consider climate and the possibility of extended power outages, which may require additional water storage.

When preparing for an emergency, it is recommended to store at least one gallon of water per person per day. However, if a family lives in a hot or dry climate, it is recommended to store more water per person per day. Additionally, if there is a family member with a medical condition that requires extra water, it is recommended to store additional water for them.

It is essential to store water properly to ensure that it is safe to consume in an emergency. Store water in clean, airtight containers that are specifically designed for water storage. Do not store water in containers that previously contained other liquids or foods, as they may contaminate the water.

Here is a story of the family dynamic and water calculation. The Johnson family consists of four hikers: Sarah, her husband Mark, and their two children, Alex and Emily. They had been planning their hiking trip in the Utah desert for months and knew that the heat would be intense. They meticulously calculated how much water they would need based on the number of family members and the length of the hike. Each member of the family carried a hydration pack and two extra bottles of water.

On the first day of the hike, they consumed approximately 4 liters of water. However, on the second day, they encountered unexpected obstacles. The trail was more difficult than they had anticipated, and the heat was relentless. Despite their careful calculations, they quickly realized that they were going through water much faster than they had anticipated.

The Johnsons had originally planned to hike for six days and had brought a total of 60 liters of water. However, by the end of the second day, they had already consumed 16 liters of water, leaving them with only 44 liters for the remaining four days. The family quickly sprang into action and made the tough decision to turn around and head back to their campsite instead of continuing on with their original plan.

Back at their campsite, the family huddled together and discussed their options. They still had several days of hiking ahead of them, but they had already gone through a large portion of their water supply. They rationed their remaining water and decided to use their filtration system to collect water from a nearby stream.

The next few days were grueling, but the Johnsons stuck to their plan. They drank only the amount of water they had calculated they needed, which was approximately 2.5 liters per day per person, even though they were all feeling thirsty and tired. They continued to use their filtration system to collect water and made sure to purify it before drinking.

Finally, on the fifth day of the hike, the Johnsons emerged from the desert, tired and sunburned, but alive. They had successfully calculated their water intake needs, rationed their water supply, and used their filtration system to collect and purify water. They had made it out of the desert, and they knew that their success was due in large part to their careful planning and attention to detail.

The Johnson family's story is a testament to the importance of calculating water needs when in a survival situation. It's not just about having enough water; it's about using it wisely and making sure there is enough on hand to last until the next water source is reached. By carefully planning their water supply and sticking to their plan, the Johnsons were able to survive the intense heat and emerge from the desert unscathed.

Water is an essential nutrient for human health and well-being. Understanding daily water requirements, the signs of dehydration, and how to calculate a family's water needs is critical to ensure being prepared for an emergency. By following these guidelines, it is easier to ensure that everyone in the family has access to safe drinking water in an emergency. Another aspect of awareness that is crucial to water supply is making sure you have created a family water plan before the next emergency occurs.

Creating a Family Water Supply Plan in an Emergency

Let's face it; water is not always the most exciting thing to drink. It can be boring to plan as well. However, when it comes to survival, we can't be too picky. So, how can we make emergency water storage more interesting? Below are a few things to consider to liven up your family water supply plan.

Have fun: One idea is to give water storage containers fun names. For example, labeling the water bottles as "H2Oasis," "Aqua la Vista," or "Water You Waiting For?" It may seem silly, but it can bring a bit of levity to an otherwise serious situation.

Family project: Another idea is to make water storage a family project. Get creative and decorate these water storage containers with fun designs or paint them in bright colors. It can be a fun way to get the whole family involved and make emergency preparedness more enjoyable.

Variation: When it comes to storing water, it's important to have a mix of different types of containers, such as large jugs, water barrels, and individual water bottles. This will help ensure that there is enough water for different situations and they can be easily transported if needed. It is also wise to have a variety of purification methods available for your family to use in an emergency. Think iodine tablets, water filtration system, boiling etc.

Location: It's also a good idea to store the water supply in a cool, dark place, such as a basement or closet. This will help prevent the growth of bacteria and keep the water fresh for a longer period. Along the location lines, it is crucial to identify emergency water sources near you such as a stored water supply, a flowing stream, a pond. With proper equipment, these could aid in your families well-being and safety in the event of a water emergency.

Conservation: Establish a water conservation plan in the event of a water shortage in your area. Guidelines of how much water each person will be allowed to use each day, as well as in which capacities, would be helpful.

Rotation: Finally, make sure to periodically rotate the water supply to keep it fresh. A good rule of thumb is to replace an emergency water supply every 6 months. One could even make it a fun family tradition to celebrate "Water Rotation Day."

Creating an emergency water supply strategy doesn't have to be boring or daunting. With a bit of humor and creativity, it can be made into a fun and engaging project for the whole family. Several of these topics will be discussed in more detail in the coming chapters, but this was a brief overview of how to create a functional family plan for emergency water supply.

PMA Toward H20 for Survival Situations (Positive Mental Attitude)

After crunching some basic numbers on a family water needs calculator, or potentially devising a plan on a spreadsheet for your family needs, it is also crucial to begin to develop a prepper's mindset toward water in a survival situation. I have a chapter dedicated to PMA in my 1st book New Prepper's Survival Bible, and also touch on it in my 2nd book Critical Nuclear War Survival Skills Guide. Attitude is THAT IMPORTANT when everything is on the line in a disaster situation or life-threatening scenario. Those that keep a level head and positive mindset typically come out ahead.

In emergency scenarios it is essential to stay positive and focused on what can actually be controlled, not wandering off mentally to all of the crazy outside factors that are outside one's control. There will be many of these outside distractions in a disaster situation, as things can "go south" rather quickly and the bad things may begin to pile up like the trash! Many people today call the act of staying present and aware of their thoughts and emotions "mindfulness". Practicing mindfulness will often reduce stress or lower anxiety. This is not a book about mindfulness, I'm simply restating what experts say on the topic.

However, along with mindfulness, there are a few more mind skills to sharpen in order to stay out in front of the pack and increase resiliency in survival. Here are a few mental skills to sharpen to keep that PMA during a water emergency.

Adaptability: The process of adjusting to new situations quickly and bouncing back from difficult situations. By being adaptable, preppers can pivot their plans and approaches when necessary, which is essential in emergency situations.

Preparedness: Maintaining a sense of preparedness involves staying organized, having a plan, and having the necessary supplies and equipment. By being prepared mentally, preppers can reduce stress and anxiety, which can improve their mental attitude.

Positive self-talk: It is crucial in a worst-case scenario event that preppers use positive language to speak to themselves. This act can improve their confidence and reduce anxiety and negative thoughts.

Gratitude: The practice of focusing on the positive things in their life. This can improve their mental attitude, reduce stress, and maintain a sense of perspective. Any clean water you have is better than no water!

By honing these positive mental attitude skills, it will increase your chances of being mentally and emotionally prepared for emergencies and disasters. This can ultimately help you maintain a level of safety and well-being in difficult situations. Yes, this applies to water as it is the #1 resource … Stay focused, stay positive, stay alive!

In a survival situation, it is critical to have access to clean drinking water. Water is essential for life, just like keeping POSITIVE thoughts are essential to living! The "survival rule of 3" comes to mind here. The rule goes like this, the average person can not go: 3 minutes without air, 3 hours without shelter, 3 days without water, or 3 weeks without food. I would add another rule, 3 seconds without hope is a killer! If a person allows themselves to mentally go down that dark path of doom and gloom in a survival situation they will often give up or even perish! They certainly will not see all the potential opportunities that are in front of them. It is so very important to engage in the here and now. Keeping that PMA increases the odds and allows them to clearly prioritize their efforts towards ensuring they have enough water to sustain themselves and their families. Here are some activities to stay engaged RIGHT NOW, that will help in the present, when dealing with a water emergency situation.

Identify potential water sources: In preparing for an emergency they should identify potential water sources in their area, such as streams, lakes, and rivers. They should also research how to locate and access these sources, and know how to purify the water to make it safe for consumption.

Stockpile water: Preppers should have a water stockpile that can sustain them and their families for a minimum of three days. This water should be stored in a clean, safe location and in containers that are specifically designed for water storage.

Develop water conservation habits: In a survival situation, it is essential to conserve water. Preppers should develop water conservation habits such as taking short showers, minimizing cooking and cleaning water usage, and using water-saving techniques for personal hygiene.

Practice water purification techniques: Preppers should practice various water purification techniques, including boiling, chemical treatment, and using water filters. It is rare that we are good at something the very first time we do it. So practice and be bad when things are good, so you have perfected it when it goes bad! They should also have the necessary equipment and supplies to purify water and know how to use them effectively. This will be discussed at length in the chapters that follow.

Plan for emergency situations: Preppers should plan for emergency situations, such as natural disasters, by having an emergency water storage plan in place. They should also be prepared to adapt and find water sources quickly if their primary sources become unavailable.

Stay informed: Preppers should stay informed about water-related news and updates in their area. This can include information about water quality, water restrictions, and potential water shortages.

Support networks: Preppers should build support networks, such as friends, family, or other preppers, to share information, resources, and emotional support. By having a support network, preppers can reduce feelings of isolation and improve their mental attitude.

Ensuring access to clean drinking water when it is not readily available, or when times are uncertain, is not something to take for granted. These mental skills and physical activities are important to consider for optimal outcomes in survival scenarios.

Here is one of my favorite true stories of pushing the limits in life, to survive even when there is no water available.

In 1994, Italian ultramarathon runner Mauro Prosperi was participating in the Marathon des Sables, a six-day ultramarathon race in Morocco that covers over 150 miles of the Sahara Desert. On the fourth day of the race, Prosperi lost his way and began running in the wrong direction. He continued to run for several hours until he realized his mistake, but by that time he was hopelessly lost in the vast expanse of the desert.

Over the next several days, Prosperi survived by drinking his own urine and eating snakes, lizards, and bats. He also found a small amount of water in a dry riverbed, but it was not enough to sustain him. Despite the harsh conditions and his rapidly deteriorating physical state, Prosperi refused to give up and kept moving in the hope of finding help.

As the days went on, Prosperi's situation grew increasingly dire. He became severely dehydrated and began experiencing hallucinations. At one point, he even considered taking his own life to end his suffering. However, he found the strength to continue, driven by a fierce determination to survive.

After ten days, Prosperi stumbled upon an abandoned Muslim shrine in Algeria. He found some supplies there, including matches, candles, and a Quran. Prosperi built a shelter and began using the candles for light and the Quran for comfort. He also used the matches to start a fire and cook the snakes and lizards he had caught.

Eventually, Prosperi regained enough strength to continue his journey. He followed the stars and the sun, moving during the cooler hours of the day and resting in the shade during the hottest part of the day. Finally, after seventeen days of wandering in the desert, he stumbled upon a military base in Algeria and was rescued.

Prosperi had lost 35 pounds during his ordeal and was severely dehydrated, but he survived. His story of survival has become a source of inspiration for endurance athletes and outdoor enthusiasts, demonstrating the importance of perseverance and resourcefulness in the face of extreme adversity. He has since become an advocate for safe and responsible wilderness travel, emphasizing the importance of carrying proper equipment and staying alert and aware of one's surroundings.

By understanding the daily water requirements of humans, the signs and symptoms of dehydration, and how to calculate family water needs, a person can create a water survival plan that will help them and their loved ones stay hydrated during an emergency situation. With a positive attitude and a well-executed plan, they will increase their chances of survival and ensure that their family has access to this essential resource when it is needed most.

Chapter 2:

Water Sources on Planet Earth

"I believe that water is the closest thing to a God we have here on Earth. We are in awe of its power and majestic beauty. We are drawn to it as if it's a magical, healing force. We gestate in water, are made of water, and need to drink water to live. We are living in water." –Alex Z. Moores

Water is the most critical resource on our planet, and access to clean and safe water is a fundamental human right. Our planet is blessed with an abundance of water, with around 71% of its surface covered in water. However, not all water sources are created equal, and access to clean and safe water remains a challenge for many people around the world. In this chapter, we will explore the various natural and man-made water sources on planet Earth and their significance to human life.

NATURAL Sources of Water

Natural water sources, such as lakes, rivers, and oceans, are essential for the survival of all living things. They provide us with water for drinking, irrigation, and sanitation. However, natural water sources are not always readily available, and factors such as drought, pollution, and climate change can impact their availability. Let's take a closer look at a few.

Streams, Rivers, and Lakes

Natural sources of water, such as streams, rivers, and lakes, are located all over the world. They are essential for human survival, providing us with drinking water, irrigation for crops, and water for sanitation. These natural water sources are often found in remote areas, away from human settlements, and are usually the result of rain and snowfall in mountainous areas.

Streams are small, flowing bodies of water that usually originate from underground springs or melting snow. They can be found in forests, meadows, and mountainous areas, and are often sources of drinking water for nearby communities.

Rivers are larger than streams and can be found in valleys and plains, where they flow towards the ocean. They are important for irrigation and hydroelectric power generation.

Lakes are large bodies of water that are surrounded by land. They are often fed by rivers and streams and provide important sources of drinking water, as well as recreational activities such as swimming and boating. These natural sources of water are vital for maintaining biodiversity, as they provide habitats for aquatic life and waterfowl.

Identifying whether the water from these natural sources is clean is crucial for human health. One way to identify if the water is clean is by observing its appearance. Clear water that is free from color and odor is usually safe to drink. However, water that appears cloudy or has an unusual color may contain harmful pollutants or bacteria.

Another way to identify if water is clean is by testing it for contamination. Testing can be done through a water testing laboratory or with water testing kits that can be purchased from hardware stores or online. These tests can detect a range of contaminants, including bacteria, viruses, and chemicals.

It is also important to consider the location of the water source. Natural water sources that are located in urban or industrial areas are more likely to be contaminated with pollutants, such as pesticides, heavy metals, and chemicals. If there is any uncertainty about the safety of a water source, it is best to avoid drinking or using it and to seek an alternative source of water.

Rainwater (Harvesting & Storing)

Rainwater is one of the most important natural sources of water on our planet, and it has been used for centuries for drinking, cooking, and cleaning. In recent years, there has been a renewed interest in harvesting rainwater for use during an emergency situation. This is because rainwater is a free and sustainable source of water that can be easily collected and stored for future use.

Rainwater harvesting involves capturing and storing rainwater that falls on roofs, gutters, and other surfaces. The collected water is then filtered and treated to make it safe for human consumption. There are a few factors to consider when planning for rainwater harvesting, including the size of the collection system, the type of storage tanks, and the quality of the water.

The first step in rainwater harvesting is to determine the amount of rainfall that can be collected from the roof or other surfaces. This will depend on the size of the roof or surface area, as well as the amount of rainfall in the area. The collected water is then diverted to a storage tank through gutters and downspouts.

The type of storage tank used for rainwater harvesting is also important. It should be made of a material that is resistant to corrosion, such as polyethylene, fiberglass, or concrete. The storage tank should be covered to prevent evaporation and contamination from insects, birds, and other animals.

The quality of the rainwater is also key. Rainwater can be contaminated with bacteria, viruses, and other pollutants, especially if it comes into contact with animal feces, bird droppings, or other contaminants. It is important to filter and treat the water to make it safe for human consumption. This can be done using a combination of physical, chemical, and biological treatment methods, depending on the quality of the water.

In an emergency situation, rainwater harvesting can provide a reliable source of water for drinking, cooking, and cleaning. It is important to plan ahead and have a sufficient amount of storage capacity to meet every need. The amount of water needed will depend on the number of people and animals that need to be supplied with water, as well as the duration of the emergency situation.

It is also important to consider the location of the collection system. It should be located away from trees and other structures that can obstruct the collection of rainwater. The collection system should also be located away from areas where there is a risk of contamination, such as septic tanks, composting toilets, and animal pens.

In conclusion, rainwater harvesting is an important strategy for sourcing and harvesting water during an emergency situation. It is a sustainable and reliable source of water that can be easily collected and stored for future use. By planning ahead and following basic guidelines for rainwater harvesting, a family can ensure that they have a sufficient supply of safe and clean water during an emergency situation.

(*BONUS*) How to Build a Rainwater harvesting system at home:

Building a rainwater harvesting system can be a great way to conserve water and reduce the reliance on municipal water supplies. Here are some general steps to consider when building a rainwater harvesting system:

Evaluate the available space: Consider the amount of space available and what type of system would be best for the needs at hand. Depending on the size of the property, a person may choose to install a small rain barrel or a larger cistern.

Determining water needs: Think about how the harvested rainwater would be used. Will it be used in irrigation, flushing toilets, or other non-potable uses? Understanding these specific water needs will help determine the size of the system needed to be built.

Select a collection surface: The collection surface is where the rainwater will be gathered. Common collection surfaces include rooftops, awnings, or other structures that can channel the rainwater to a downspout.

Install a gutter system: To collect the rainwater from the roof, one would need to install a gutter system if not installed already. This will direct the rainwater into a downspout and into the collection system.

Install a storage container: The rainwater will be stored in a container such as a rain barrel or cistern. Make sure to choose a container that is made for storing water, and that has a secure lid to keep debris and insects out.

Install a filtration system: It's important to filter the collected rainwater before it is used. This can be done by installing a filtration system such as a mesh screen or a more complex filtration system.

Install a distribution system: Once the rainwater has been filtered and stored, it will need to be distributed to where it will be used. This may involve installing a pump, pipes, and valves to direct the water to where it is needed.

Consider the local regulations: Be sure to check with local government guidelines to ensure that the project follows any regulations regarding rainwater harvesting.

These are some general steps to consider when building a rainwater harvesting system. Depending on specific needs, this project may need to be slightly modified so possibly consult with a professional for guidance.

Groundwater

Groundwater can be an important source of water for consumption in a survival situation, as it can often be more reliable than surface water sources, such as streams or lakes, which can be impacted by drought, pollution, or other factors. Here are some reasons why groundwater can be a viable source of water, as well as ways to harvest and distribute this water, and how to properly filter it if needed for an emergency.

Importance of groundwater:

Groundwater can be a more reliable source of water, as it is less impacted by seasonal variations, drought, or surface pollution.

Groundwater can often be of higher quality than surface water, as it is naturally filtered through soil and rock.

Groundwater can be accessed through wells or springs, which can provide a consistent supply of water over time.

Harvesting and distributing groundwater:

To access groundwater, a well can be dug or drilled into the ground to reach the aquifer, which is the underground layer of water-bearing rock or soil.

A hand pump or other mechanical system can be used to draw the water up from the well, and then distributed to where it is needed.

If a natural spring is present, the water can be collected using a container or piping system to bring it to where it is needed.

Filtering groundwater:

While groundwater is generally of higher quality than surface water, it can still contain contaminants, such as bacteria, viruses, or chemicals, that can make it unsafe to drink.

Filtration can be achieved through various methods, such as using a portable water filter, a ceramic filter, or a sand filter.

Boiling the water can also be an effective way to kill most bacteria and viruses, although it may not remove all contaminants.

When harvesting and filtering groundwater for consumption, it is important to follow proper sanitation and hygiene practices to avoid contamination. For example, the well or spring should be properly sealed and protected to prevent surface runoff and animal waste from entering the water supply. Additionally, any containers used to transport or store the water should be clean and disinfected to prevent contamination.

Natural Springs

Natural springs are a valuable source of freshwater for many communities around the world. Springs occur when underground water that has been stored in an aquifer flows up to the surface due to natural pressure, creating a natural outlet for fresh water. Springs can be found in a variety of geological settings, including volcanic areas, limestone formations, and mountainous regions, and can vary in size, flow rate, and water quality. Here are some of the different types of natural springs found on Earth, and how humans can use them for clean water sources.

Types of Usable Springs for Clean Water Sources

Artesian springs: Artesian springs are found in areas where groundwater is stored in an underground aquifer that is confined between layers of impermeable rock. The pressure from the water in the confined aquifer causes it to flow up to the surface, creating an artesian spring. These springs are often high in quality, as the water is naturally filtered through the surrounding rock formations.

Limestone springs: Limestone springs are found in areas where the underlying rock is made up of porous limestone that allows water to flow through it. The water that emerges from limestone springs is typically very high in minerals and can have a distinct taste due to the dissolved calcium and magnesium ions. Many communities use limestone springs as a source of drinking water, but the high mineral content can cause issues with hard water and mineral buildup.

Volcanic springs: Volcanic springs are found in areas where the underlying rock has been formed from volcanic activity. The water that emerges from these springs is typically very hot and often contains minerals like sulfur, which can create a distinct odor. While the high temperatures can make it difficult to use volcanic springs for drinking water, they can be used for geothermal power generation or therapeutic hot springs.

Mountain springs: Mountain springs are found in areas where the underlying rock formations have been exposed due to erosion. The water that emerges from these springs is often very pure, as it has been naturally filtered through the surrounding rock formations. Many communities rely on mountain springs for their drinking water, but they can be vulnerable to pollution from surface runoff or other sources.

Protecting & Conserving Springs for Years of Use

In order to use natural springs as a source of clean water, humans need to take steps to protect them from pollution and maintain their flow rates. Here are some ways to do this:

Protect the watershed: The watershed surrounding the spring needs to be protected from activities that could pollute the water, such as agriculture, mining, or other land use activities. This can be achieved through careful land management practices, such as reducing pesticide use, planting cover crops, and reducing soil erosion.

Monitor the flow rate: The flow rate of the spring needs to be monitored to ensure that it is not being overused or depleted. This can be achieved through regular measurement of the water levels and flow rates, as well as careful management of water use.

Protect the spring outlet: The outlet of the spring needs to be protected from pollution and disturbance, such as from construction or other human activities. This can be achieved through careful management of the surrounding land use and the installation of protective barriers.

In summary, natural springs are a valuable source of freshwater for many communities around the world, and there are many different types of springs with varying water quality and mineral content. To use natural springs as a source of clean water, humans need to take steps to protect the surrounding watershed, monitor the flow rate, and protect the outlet from pollution and disturbance. With careful management, natural springs can provide a sustainable and reliable source of fresh water for many communities.

Man-made Sources of Water

Man-made water sources, such as reservoirs, wells, and desalination plants, have become increasingly important in meeting the growing demand for water. These sources are the result of human ingenuity and innovation, and they play a crucial role in ensuring that people have access to clean and safe water.

Wells

Wells are one of the oldest man-made sources of water. They have been in use for thousands of years to provide access to groundwater for drinking, irrigation, and other purposes. A well is a vertical shaft or hole dug into the ground to reach an aquifer, which is a layer of permeable rock or sediment that holds water. Water can then be pumped or drawn out of the well for use.

There are various types of water wells, including dug wells, driven wells, drilled wells, and bored wells. Each type of well has its own advantages and disadvantages, depending on factors such as the depth of the water table, the soil and rock types, and the desired well capacity. Here is a brief overview of each type:

Types of Wells

Dug wells: These are the simplest type of well, typically dug by hand or with a backhoe. They are generally shallow, with depths ranging from a few feet to 30 feet. Dug wells are typically used for domestic purposes and can provide water from shallow aquifers.

Driven wells: These are typically used in areas with shallow water tables and soft soil. A small-diameter pipe is driven into the ground with a special driving point or well point, and a screen is added to allow water to enter the well.

Bored wells: These are similar to dug wells, but are typically deeper and drilled with a machine. They are often used for larger water supplies or for commercial and industrial purposes.

Drilled wells: These are the most common type of well, and are typically drilled by a professional drilling company using specialized equipment. Drilled wells can be deep, up to several hundred feet, and can access deep aquifers that provide large quantities of water.

How to Build a Dug Well at Home (Bonus!)

Here is a quick step-by-step guide for building a simple dug well at home:

Choose a location: Choose a location that is away from sources of contamination, such as septic systems or chemical storage areas.

Dig the well: Use a shovel or backhoe to dig a hole in the ground to the desired depth, making sure to remove any loose soil or debris.

Line the well: Line the walls of the well with concrete, bricks, or stones to prevent collapse and to improve water quality.

Add a screen: Add a screen at the bottom of the well to allow water to enter while keeping out debris and sediment.

Install a pump: Install a hand or electric pump at the top of the well to draw water from the well.

Cover the well: Cover the well with a protective cap or lid to prevent contamination and to ensure safety.

It is important to note that building a well can be a complex and potentially dangerous process, and it is recommended to consult a professional well driller or contractor for any significant well construction projects.

Pro's & Con's of Wells

Wells have several advantages over other sources of water. They are relatively easy to construct and can provide a reliable and consistent supply of water. They are also relatively inexpensive to maintain and can be a more sustainable source of water compared to surface water sources that can be impacted by drought, pollution, and other environmental factors.

However, wells also have some disadvantages. They can be susceptible to contamination from surface runoff, animal waste, and other sources. They can also be impacted by overuse, which can deplete the aquifer and cause the well to run dry. Additionally, the quality of well water can vary depending on the location and geology of the aquifer.

Overall, wells can be an important source of water for communities and individuals, but it is important to ensure that they are properly constructed, maintained, and monitored to protect both the quality and quantity of the water supply.

Ponds and Reservoirs

Reservoirs and ponds are man-made sources of water that are used to store and supply water for various purposes. Reservoirs are typically larger than ponds and can hold significant amounts of water, while ponds are generally smaller and used for more localized purposes.

Reservoirs are usually constructed by building a dam across a river or stream, creating a large, artificial lake behind it. The stored water can then be used for drinking water, irrigation, hydroelectric power generation, and recreational activities. Reservoirs can be an effective way to store water and provide a reliable water source, but they can also have negative impacts on the environment, such as altering river flows, disrupting fish habitats, and reducing downstream water quality.

Ponds, on the other hand, are usually created by excavating a depression in the ground and lining it with materials such as clay or concrete. Ponds can be used for a variety of purposes, including irrigation, livestock watering, aquaculture, and recreational activities. However, ponds can also be a source of water quality issues if they are not properly maintained or if they become contaminated by runoff or other sources of pollution.

Overall, reservoirs and ponds can be important man-made sources of water, but it is important to consider their potential impacts on the environment and to properly manage and maintain them to ensure that they provide a safe and sustainable water source for their intended purposes.

Water Tanks

Water tanks are a man-made source of water that are used to store and supply water for a variety of purposes, such as drinking, irrigation, firefighting, and industrial processes. Water tanks can range in size from small, above-ground containers to large, underground storage tanks that hold millions of gallons of water.

Water tanks can be made of various materials, including concrete, steel, fiberglass, and plastic. Each material has its own advantages and disadvantages, depending on factors such as cost, durability, and environmental impact. In addition, water tanks can be equipped with a variety of features, such as pumps, filters, and sensors, to improve water quality, control flow, and monitor usage.

One of the key advantages of water tanks is their ability to store water for times of drought or other water supply disruptions. They can also be used to store and distribute water from other sources, such as rainwater, groundwater, or surface water.

However, there are also some disadvantages to using water tanks as a source of water. For example, the initial cost of installing a water tank can be high, and ongoing maintenance and repair can also be costly. In addition, water tanks can be susceptible to contamination from sediment, bacteria, and other pollutants, and it is important to properly maintain and clean the tanks to prevent water quality issues.

Overall, water tanks can be an important man-made source of water, providing a reliable and sustainable water supply for various purposes. However, it is important to consider the environmental and economic impacts of installing and maintaining water tanks, and to properly manage and monitor them to ensure that they provide safe and high-quality water.

Swimming Pools

Really? Yup. Swimming pools are a man-made source of water that can potentially be used in emergency situations to provide a source of water for drinking, sanitation, and other essential needs. However, there are several important considerations and precautions that must be taken before using pool water in this way.

First, it is important to note that swimming pool water is treated with chemicals, such as chlorine, to keep it clean and free of bacteria and other pathogens. These chemicals can be harmful if ingested in large quantities, and can cause skin and eye irritation. Therefore, it is important to filter and treat the pool water to remove these chemicals before using it for drinking or other purposes.

Second, swimming pool water may also contain other contaminants, such as dirt, debris, and other pollutants, that can affect its quality and safety. It is important to properly filter and treat the water to remove these contaminants, and to regularly monitor the water quality to ensure that it remains safe to use.

Drinking saltwater from a pool is not recommended, as it can be harmful to human health due to its high salt content. Ingesting salt water can cause dehydration and electrolyte imbalances, which can lead to further health complications.

However, if one finds themselves in a desperate survival situation where there is no other source of freshwater available and they need to drink salt water to survive, there are a few methods that can help make the salt water safer to drink.

One method is to use a solar still, which can help remove the salt and other impurities from the water. To make a solar still, dig a hole in the ground near the pool and place a container in the center. Cover the hole with a clear plastic sheet and weight down the edges with rocks or other objects. As the sun heats up the water in the hole, it will evaporate and condense on the underside of the plastic sheet, collecting in the container.

Another method is to use a desalination kit, which can remove the salt and other impurities from the water through a process of reverse osmosis or distillation. Desalination kits are available for purchase, but they can be expensive and may not be readily available in an emergency situation.

In any case, it is important to remember that drinking saltwater should only be done as a last resort and under extreme circumstances. It is always best to seek out other sources of freshwater, such as rainwater, groundwater, or other natural sources, whenever possible.

Finally, swimming pool water may not be a sustainable or long-term solution for emergency water needs, as it may be depleted quickly and may not be replenished. It is important to have other sources of water available, such as stored water or rainwater collection, to ensure a reliable and sustainable water supply.

In summary, while swimming pools can potentially be used as a man-made source of water in emergency situations, it is important to take proper precautions and to consider the quality and sustainability of the water supply. It is also important to consult with experts and authorities before using swimming pool water in this way to ensure that it is safe and appropriate for the intended use.

Community Water Sources

In emergency situations, having access to safe and reliable sources of water is crucial for survival. In many communities, there are man-made water sources that can be used in such situations. Some of the common types of community water sources include:

Municipal water systems: These are water treatment and distribution systems that are owned and managed by local governments or utility companies. They typically rely on surface water or groundwater sources and use a variety of treatment methods to remove contaminants and ensure that the water is safe to drink.

Community water storage tanks: These are large water storage tanks that are typically used in rural or remote communities where access to municipal water systems is limited. Community water storage tanks can provide a reliable source of water in emergency situations, but it is important to properly maintain and treat the water to prevent contamination.

Community Irrigation systems: A man-made channel or pipeline that brings water from a distant source, such as a river or lake, to irrigate farmland or supply water to a community. These may not be accessible in urban areas, more popular in rural settings.

To use these community water sources in emergency situations, it is important to take the following steps:

Ensure that the water is safe to drink by testing it regularly and following proper treatment and filtration methods.

Store the water in clean, secure containers that are free from contaminants.

Use the water for essential needs such as drinking, cooking, and hygiene, and conserve it as much as possible to ensure a sustainable supply.

Properly maintain and monitor the community water sources to ensure that they continue to provide safe and reliable water in emergency situations.

Man-made community water sources can be valuable sources of water in emergency situations, but it is important to properly treat, store, and maintain the water to ensure that it is safe to drink and use. By taking these precautions, communities can ensure a reliable and sustainable water supply in times of need.

Factors to Consider When Choosing Water Sources in a Survival Situation

Choosing a water source in a survival situation or water emergency can be a task that's just guaranteed to put a smile on one's face and a spring in one's step, right? Well, maybe not, but we can still approach it with a sense of humor.

When it comes to choosing a water source, there are a few important factors to consider. First, the source needs to be reliable. It would be unfortunate to trek halfway across the desert to reach a well that's dried up. Another scenario would be discovering a creek that's only running for a few hours a day. Make sure the water source can be depended on. Multiple water sources is a very good idea when considering this in terms of an emergency event. The "outside the box" ideas or locations will usually be where less people are, and trust me people will be desperate, so use your brain for any advantage.

Next, choose a source that's clean. If one is going to be drinking the water, one doesn't want to be getting sick from it. So, avoid stagnant water that's likely to be full of bacteria and other nasty things. And definitely steer clear of anything that looks like it's been touched by human or animal waste. That's just gross.

Third, one wants a source that's easy to access. One doesn't want to be doing acrobatics to reach the water. One wants to be able to get to it quickly and easily. So, make sure the source chosen is one that can be accessed without too much trouble.

Finally, one wants a source that's plentiful. One doesn't want to be struggling to get enough water to meet one's needs. One wants a source that's going to provide all the water needed to survive.

Now, once a water source has been found, what does one do? Well, first off, make sure the water is being collected in a clean container. No one wants to be drinking out of a dirty, bacteria-filled bottle. That's just gross, and dangerous! Second, treat the water before drinking it. Boiling is a good way to kill off any bacteria, or water purification tablets can be used if they are available. Pouring the water through a filtration unit is an option, or even pouring mucky water through a sock with some charcoal in it from last night's fire like Bear Grylls does is better than nothing!

Choosing a water source in a survival situation or water emergency can be a daunting task, but with a little bit of humor and common sense, one can find a source that's reliable, clean, easy to access, and plentiful. With a little bit of preparation, that yucky water can be turned into a refreshing drink that will keep one going until help arrives. Cheers to that!

In this chapter, we discussed in detail the types of water sources that may be encountered during an emergency situation. In the following chapter I will highlight the significance of water purification. Even if a seemingly reliable, clean, and plentiful water

source is found, it is still crucial to purify the water before consumption. The next chapter will delve into the details of water purification.

Chapter 3:

Water Purifying Methods

"If there is magic on this planet, it is contained in water." —Loren Eiseley

Water is essential for our survival. This phrase has been stated several times already, and the intentional use of redundancy is stressing the crucial importance of the topic at hand. Water is necessary for our body's proper functioning and helps regulate our body temperature, aids in digestion, and eliminates waste. However, not all water sources are safe to consume, and in emergency situations, when access to clean water is limited, one must find ways to make it safe for consumption.

Importance of Water Purification

Purification is the process of removing or destroying any harmful contaminants or pathogens that may be present in the water. This includes bacteria, viruses, and parasites, as well as any chemicals or toxins that may be present.

Purification can be done through a variety of methods, including boiling, filtration, and the use of water purification tablets or drops. Each method has its own advantages and disadvantages, and it is important to choose the method that is best suited for the specific situation.

Purification is essential to ensure that the water being consumed is safe and free from harmful contaminants that can lead to illness or disease. Properly purifying the water can help reduce the risk of sickness and ensure that individuals remain healthy and hydrated during emergency situations. Let's now look at several water purifying methods in more depth.

Boiling

One of the most effective and reliable methods of purifying water is boiling. Boiling water is a simple yet effective method of water purification. It involves heating water to its boiling point, which kills most of the bacteria, viruses, and parasites that may be present in the water. The World Health Organization (WHO) recommends boiling water for at least 1 minute to ensure that it is safe for consumption. In a natural environment, this may vary slightly. The Wilderness Medical Society and the CDC (Center for Disease Control) agree that boiling water for an average of 2 to 3 minutes at temperatures of 140-160 degrees Fahrenheit is sufficient to kill Water Borne Pathogens.

To purify water using boiling, follow these steps:

Collect the water: Find a source of water that is as clean as possible. If possible, choose flowing water sources such as a river or stream rather than stagnant sources. Collect water in a clean container, making sure not to contaminate it in the process.

Filter the water: If the water is murky or has visible impurities, it is essential to filter it before boiling. Do this by using a cloth, coffee filter, or even a piece of clothing to remove large particles from the water.

Boil the water: Place the water in a pot and heat it on a stove or over an open fire. Once the water reaches a rolling boil, let it continue boiling for at least one minute. 99.9% of water borne microorganisms can be killed at five minutes of exposure to 149 F/65 C temperatures of water. In high altitude locations, the water may need to boil for longer as the boiling point is lower at higher elevations.

Let the water cool: Once water has boiled, remove it from the heat and let it cool. Avoid touching the water or using dirty containers or utensils, as this can contaminate it.

Store the water: Once the water has cooled, transfer it to a clean container with a tight-fitting lid. Adding a pinch of salt will improve the taste of the water.

It is worth noting that boiling water may not remove all contaminants from the water, such as chemicals or heavy metals. In such cases, it is best to seek alternative water sources or use a more advanced water treatment method.

Boiling water is a reliable and cost-effective method of water purification that has been used for centuries. It is a simple method that requires only basic equipment and can be done almost anywhere. However, it is essential to ensure that the water has reached a rolling boil for at least 1 minute to kill most of the harmful bacteria and viruses.

Here are some statistics and facts about boiling water:

- According to the World Health Organization (WHO), boiling water for at least 1 minute can kill most of the bacteria, viruses, and parasites that may be present in the water.

- The Center for Disease Control and Prevention (CDC) recommends boiling water for 1 minute to make it safe to drink, or 3 minutes at higher elevations above 6,562 feet (2,000 meters).

- In 2018, a study by the United Nations Children's Fund (UNICEF) and the World Health Organization (WHO) found that 2.2 billion people around the world lack access to safe drinking water

- Unsafe drinking water can cause waterborne diseases such as cholera, typhoid fever, and diarrhea, which can be deadly, especially for children and people with weakened immune systems.

- Boiling water is one of the oldest and most effective methods of water purification, dating back to ancient times when it was used to make water safe for consumption.

In the wild, access to clean water is often limited, and being able to purify water is critical to staying hydrated and alive. One of the most remarkable real-life stories of surviving dehydration and lack of water in the wild is the story of Aron Ralston, an American mountaineer who became trapped in a remote canyon in Utah.

In 2006, a hiker named Aron Ralston was canyoneering alone in Blue John Canyon in southeastern Utah. While rappelling down a slot canyon, a boulder dislodged and crushed his right arm, pinning him against the canyon wall. He was unable to move and was stuck there for 5 days with only a limited supply of water.

Ralston knew that he had to conserve his water as much as possible if he wanted to survive. He rationed his water carefully, drinking only small sips to stay hydrated. But as the days passed, he began to run out of water and knew that he needed to find more.

After several failed attempts to free himself, Ralston decided to take drastic measures. He used a pocket knife to amputate his right arm below the elbow, in order to free himself from the boulder. Yes, you read that correctly. He then rappelled down the canyon with 1 mangled arm, and hiked several miles before coming across a small pool of stagnant water. Ralston knew that the water was not safe to drink, but he had no other option. He used a water bottle to scoop up the water and found a way to start a fire to boil the water, making it safe to drink.

Ralston's determination to survive and his resourcefulness in finding a way to make the water safe to drink saved his life. He was eventually rescued and his story of survival became the subject of the book *"Between a Rock and a Hard Place,"* which was later adapted into the film *"127 Hours."*

Ralston's story is a powerful reminder of the importance of being prepared and resourceful in the face of extreme survival situations. His will to live and his quick thinking in finding a way to make the contaminated water safe to drink are a testament to the human spirit and the will to survive against all odds.

When in a survival situation and access to clean water is limited, boiling water is an effective way to purify it. Remember to collect the water from a clean source, filter it if necessary, bring it to a rolling boil, let it boil for at least 1 minute, let it cool, and store it in a clean container. By following these steps, one can ensure that the water is safe for consumption and this will help them stay hydrated and healthy. In a life altering survival story such as Aron Ralston's, he was able to find the inner strength to make it back home safely and has since shared his story with millions to raise awareness about the importance of clean water and the need to be prepared for emergencies when venturing into the great outdoors.

Physical Methods to Purify Water - How to Turn Mud into Magic

Water is the source of life, but not all water is created equal. In fact, much of the water we encounter in the wild is downright dirty. So what do we do when we're parched, but the only water source nearby looks like a mud puddle after a rainstorm? Fear not, my friends, for in this chapter we will explore the wonderful world of water purification!

First things first, let's talk about sedimentation. This is the process of letting the water sit still and waiting for the heavier particles to sink to the bottom. But in the case of water, the goal is to remove the sediment and other large particles that can make a human sick or just give the water a funky taste. So, find 2 containers if possible, preferably 1 with 1 a lid, fill it with water, and wait. Depending on how dirty the water is, there may be a little wait, but patience is a virtue in this case. And let's be real, sometimes waiting for a miracle to happen is the only option we've got. Once the water has settled, carefully pour the clear water into the 2nd clean container, being careful not to stir up the sediment at the bottom.

Filtration

Next up, filtration. This is the process of passing water through a filter to remove impurities. In water purification, we have a few options for filtration, including screening, skimming, dipping, and flocculation.

Screening involves passing the water through a fine mesh, like a piece of cloth, to remove larger particles such as leaves, twigs, or pebbles. This method is commonly used in emergency situations when other filtration methods are not available.

Skimming water is the process of using a spoon or other tool (cloth or paper towel) to remove floating particles from the surface of the water. This can often mean oil or grease extraction as well. Visible contaminants will be easy to remove this way, however it may not remove bacteria or viruses.

Dipping (ladling) means simply scooping up cleaner water from the top of a container, being careful not to stir up the sediment at the bottom. Note if the water is stirred up, this situation is reversed. Start by removing the floating debris from the surface of the water with a ladle, and the water remaining would be cleaner water.

Finally, flocculation involves adding a substance, or chemical, to the water that causes the impurities to clump together (or floc) and sink to the bottom, making them easier to remove. It's like gathering all the bad apples in one basket just to throw them away.

When it comes to water purification, there are many methods available to us, and it's important to be familiar with as many as possible. From sedimentation and filtration to ladling or even boiling, there's a solution for every situation. Please remember, the key to successful water purification is patience, attention to detail, and a healthy sense of humor. Because let's be real, sometimes life throws us a muddy puddle to drink from, but with the right methods and attitude, we can turn that mud into magic. So go forth, my friends, and conquer thirst, one purified sip at a time with any of the above mentioned skills!

Chemical Methods of Purification- Making Water Safe, One Chemical at a Time

Water is a life-sustaining resource, but it can also be a source of harm if contaminated. Bacteria, viruses, parasites, and heavy metals can all find their way into our water sources, making them unsafe to drink. In this section we'll explore the most common chemical methods of water purification, from chlorination to adsorption, to help better understand how they work and what they can do to make drinking water safe.

Chlorination: The Classic Choice

When thinking of water purification, the first thing that comes to mind is probably chlorination. This classic chemical method has been used for over a century to purify drinking water. Chlorine is a powerful disinfectant that can kill bacteria and viruses, but it's important to use the right amount. Too little and the water won't be safe, too much and it can be harmful to humans. The amount of chlorine needed to make water drinkable depends on the specific situation, including the level of contamination and the type of microorganisms present. The general guideline is to use around 0.2 to 1.0 parts per million (ppm) of free chlorine to disinfect water. However, the exact dosage should be determined by a water treatment professional or calculated using a chlorine residual test kit.

As for how long the chlorination process takes, it can vary depending on the specific system being used. In general, the chlorine should be allowed to remain in contact with the water for at least 30 minutes to ensure proper disinfection. However, in some cases, a longer contact time may be necessary. After this contact time, the water should be tested to ensure that it has been properly disinfected and that the chlorine level has returned to a safe level for drinking.

Ozonation: Ozone's Not Just for the Ozone Layer

Ozonation is a newer method of water purification that has gained popularity in recent years. Ozone, a form of oxygen that has 3 atoms instead of 2, is an incredibly powerful oxidant. When added to water, it can destroy bacteria, viruses, and other contaminants. Plus, it has the added bonus of leaving the water smelling like a fresh, mountain breeze. There are different ways to use ozone to purify water, and some of the methods include:

Ozone Generators: There are various brands of ozone generators available on the market that can be used for water treatment. These generators create ozone gas that is then injected into the water supply to disinfect it.

Ozone Water Purification Systems: These are whole-house water treatment systems that use ozone to disinfect water at the point of entry into a home. They can be installed by a professional plumber and are available from various manufacturers.

Portable Ozone Water Purifiers: There are also portable water purifiers that use ozone to disinfect water. These are typically small devices that can be used to purify water on camping trips or in emergency situations.

When using ozonation to purify water, it's essential to follow the manufacturer's instructions carefully. In general, the process involves injecting ozone gas into the water supply and allowing it to react for a certain period of time. The amount of ozone needed will depend on the level of contamination in the water and the volume of water being treated. It's also important to note that ozone can be harmful to human health if not used properly, so it's crucial to follow all safety guidelines when using an ozonation system. Just don't go overboard and create a hole in the ozone layer, please!

Coagulation and Ion Exchange: The Dynamic Duo

Coagulation and ion exchange are two chemical methods that are often used together to purify water. Coagulation is the process of adding a chemical to water to make small particles stick together and form larger ones, which can then be filtered out. Ion exchange, on the other hand, uses a resin to remove ions from water. Both methods are highly effective in removing heavy metals, minerals, and other impurities from water, making it safe to drink.

Here are some different kinds of coagulation and ion exchange methods:

Coagulation

Aluminum sulfate (alum) coagulation: This method uses alum, a chemical compound that attracts and clumps together dirt and other particles in the water, making them easier to remove through filtration.

Ferric chloride coagulation: Ferric chloride is a coagulant that is often used in conjunction with alum. This method is especially effective at removing dissolved organic matter from water.

PAC (polyaluminum chloride) coagulation: PAC is a type of coagulant that is often used in municipal water treatment plants. It can be effective at removing a wide range of contaminants from water.

Ion Exchange

Cation exchange: This method involves the removal of positively charged ions (such as calcium, magnesium, and iron) from water by exchanging them for hydrogen ions.

Anion exchange: This method involves the removal of negatively charged ions (such as chloride, sulfate, and nitrate) from water by exchanging them for hydroxide ions.

Mixed bed ion exchange: This method involves the use of both cation and anion exchange resins in a single treatment step to remove both positively and negatively charged ions from water.

It's important to note that coagulation and ion exchange are typically used in larger-scale water treatment facilities, rather than in individual survival situations. However, knowledge of these methods can be useful in emergency situations where other water treatment options are not available.

Reverse Osmosis: Don't Judge a Process by Its Name

Reverse osmosis might sound like a complicated process, but it's actually pretty simple. It involves using a semi-permeable membrane to filter out impurities from water. The membrane allows water molecules to pass through, but it blocks larger molecules like bacteria and viruses. Reverse osmosis is highly effective at removing salt, minerals, and other impurities from water, making it safe to drink. We have an RO system in our home and it makes the drinkable well water tasty! (or tasteless I suppose?)

Here are some different kinds of reverse osmosis options and their benefits:

Portable Reverse Osmosis Filters: These small, portable filters can be used to purify water in the field or during emergency situations. They typically use a hand pump to force water through a semipermeable membrane that removes contaminants.

Under-Sink Reverse Osmosis Systems: These systems are designed to be installed under a kitchen sink or in a small workspace, and can be used to purify drinking water for daily use. They typically consist of a pre-filter, reverse osmosis membrane, and post-filter.

Whole-House Reverse Osmosis Systems: These systems are designed to be installed at the point of entry for a home's water supply, providing purified water for all uses throughout the home. They typically consist of multiple stages of filtration, including pre-filters, reverse osmosis membranes, and post-filters.

Benefits of Reverse Osmosis

Here are a few benefits of reverse osmosis with water.

Effective Removal of Contaminants: Reverse osmosis is highly effective at removing a wide range of contaminants from water, including bacteria, viruses, heavy metals, and other toxins.

Easy to Use: Many reverse osmosis systems are designed to be easy to use and require little maintenance. Depending on the size of your system, the filters last quite a long time before needing to be replaced.

Energy Efficient: Many reverse osmosis systems use minimal amounts of energy, making them a more sustainable option for water purification.

It's important to note that reverse osmosis systems can be expensive, particularly larger-scale systems designed for whole-house treatment. However, in a survival situation where access to clean water is critical, the benefits of reverse osmosis can be significant.

Adsorption: Just Like a Sponge

Adsorption is a physical method of water purification that uses activated carbon to remove impurities. Activated carbon is like a sponge that can absorb small impurities from water. It's highly effective at removing chemicals, pesticides, and other contaminants from water, but it's important to replace the carbon filter regularly to ensure it's still working at its best.

Here are some different kinds of activated carbon options and their benefits for purifying water in a survival situation:

Granular Activated Carbon (GAC): GAC is a form of activated carbon that is available in granular form, making it ideal for use in water treatment applications. GAC is effective at removing a wide range of contaminants, including chlorine, pesticides, and other organic chemicals.

Powdered Activated Carbon (PAC): PAC is a finely ground form of activated carbon that is often used in water treatment applications due to its high surface area and adsorption capacity. PAC is effective at removing a wide range of contaminants, including heavy metals, pesticides, and other organic chemicals.

Activated Carbon Filters: These filters use activated carbon to remove contaminants from water as it passes through the filter.

Activated carbon filters are available in a range of sizes and configurations, making them suitable for use in a variety of applications.

Benefits of Adsorption

Here are a few benefits of adsorption with water.

Cost Effective: Activated carbon can be a cost-effective way to purify water, particularly when compared to other treatment options such as distillation.

Safe and Environmentally Friendly: Activated carbon is a safe and environmentally friendly water treatment option, as it does not produce harmful byproducts or waste.

Effective Removal of Contaminants: Activated carbon is also highly effective at removing a wide range of contaminants from water, including organic chemicals, heavy metals, and other toxins.

It's important to note that activated carbon may not be effective at removing all contaminants from water, particularly those that are dissolved or inorganic. However, in a survival situation where access to clean water is critical, activated carbon can be a valuable tool for purifying water.

The world of water purification is vast and complex, but with the right knowledge and tools, it is not difficult to make sure water is safe to drink in almost any situation. From chlorination to adsorption, there are a variety of chemical methods available to make water safe. Just remember to always use the correct amount of chemical, and if there is any doubt, leave it to the experts.

Other Purification Methods

Welcome to the section on "Other" Water Purification Methods! In addition to the physical and chemical methods we've discussed in previous parts of the book, there are several other ways to purify water in a survival situation. Some of these methods may seem a little unconventional, but they can be highly effective when used correctly.

Ultraviolet (UV) Purification

UV purification is a water treatment method that uses ultraviolet light to kill bacteria, viruses, and other microorganisms that may be present in water. UV radiation disrupts the DNA of microorganisms, preventing them from reproducing and making them unable to cause infection. There are several common UV water purification items that are available for purchase. Here are a few examples:

SteriPen: This is a small handheld device that uses UV-C light to purify water. It can be used to treat up to 16 ounces of water at a time and can purify 8,000 liters of water before the lamp needs to be replaced.

LARQ Bottle: This is a water bottle that uses UV-C LED technology to purify water. It can purify up to 99.99% of harmful bacteria and viruses in just 60 seconds. The bottle is rechargeable and can be used to purify up to 5,000 cycles before the battery needs to be charged.

UV Water Purification Pens: These are pens that emit UV light and can be used to purify water. They are small and lightweight, making them perfect for backpacking and camping trips. They are effective at purifying bacteria and viruses and are easy to use.

Katadyn SteriPEN Aqua: This is a small, handheld UV water purifier that is designed for use on-the-go. It can be used to treat up to 50 liters of water and is effective at purifying bacteria and viruses.

These are just a few examples of the many different UV water purification items that are available for purchase. It's important to research and then choose a product that meets specific needs and requirements for the situation.

While UV purification may seem like a high-tech solution to water purification, it's actually quite simple to use. Portable UV water purifiers are available that can be powered by batteries or solar energy, making them ideal for use in remote locations. Simply place the purifier in a container of water, turn it on, and wait for the UV light to do its job.

Solar Disinfection (SOD)

If access to a UV water purifier is difficult, there's another way to use the power of the sun to purify water: solar disinfection (SOD). SOD involves filling a clear plastic bottle with water and leaving it in direct sunlight for several hours. The UV radiation in sunlight kills bacteria and viruses, making the water safe to drink. Below are several common solar disinfection items that are available for water purification.

SODIS Bottles: SODIS (Solar Water Disinfection) is a simple, low-cost method of water purification that involves filling clear plastic bottles with water and then exposing them to sunlight for several hours. SODIS bottles are widely available and can be purchased online or in stores. They are lightweight and easy to use, making them a popular choice for backpackers and hikers.

Solar Disinfection Bags: These are specially designed bags that are made from a clear, durable material that allows sunlight to pass through. They can be used to purify large volumes of water and are ideal for emergency situations or for use in areas where clean drinking water is not readily available. They are lightweight and portable, making them easy to carry.

Solar Still: This is a more complex device that uses the power of the sun to distill water. It involves filling a container with contaminated water and then placing it inside a larger container that has a clear plastic cover. As the sun heats the water, it evaporates and then condenses on the inside of the plastic cover, leaving behind any contaminants. The purified water can then be collected in a separate container.

Some benefits of using solar disinfection methods for water purification include:

Low cost: Many solar disinfection methods are low-cost or even free, making them accessible to people who might not be able to afford more advanced purification methods.

Environmentally friendly: Solar disinfection methods don't require any chemicals or energy sources other than the sun, making them an environmentally friendly option for water purification.

Widely available: SODIS bottles and other solar disinfection methods are widely available and can be purchased online or in stores, making them accessible to people all over the world. Plus, that large orange ball in the sky that warms our planet is out most days and can be used for many purposes while you are in nature.

While SOD may not be as effective as UV purification, it can be a simple and low-cost way to purify water in a survival situation. Just make sure to use a clear plastic bottle, as colored or opaque bottles can block the UV radiation from the sun.

Biological Purification

Biological water purification methods involve using living organisms to remove contaminants from water. Two common biological purification methods are biofiltration and phytoremediation.

Biofiltration involves using bacteria to break down and remove contaminants from water. In a biofilter, water is passed through a bed of material that contains bacteria, such as sand or gravel. The bacteria in the bed break down organic matter and remove harmful contaminants, such as ammonia and nitrate.

Phytoremediation involves using plants to remove contaminants from water. Certain plants, such as water hyacinths and cattails, are highly effective at absorbing and removing pollutants from water. In a survival situation, creating a phytoremediation system can be done by placing a container of water near a patch of these plants and allowing the plants to absorb the contaminants from the water.

While biological purification methods may not be as quick or effective as some physical or chemical methods, they can be highly sustainable and low-cost solutions to water purification.

While physical and chemical methods are often the go-to solutions for water purification in survival situations, it's important to remember that there are other ways to make water safe to drink. Ultraviolet purification, solar disinfection, and biological purification methods can all be.

highly effective when used correctly. And in a survival situation, it's important to have as many tools in the toolkit as possible. So keep these "other" water purification methods in mind, and stay safe out there!

Portable - Water Filters & Purifiers

When it comes to surviving in the great outdoors, having access to clean drinking water is a top priority. While boiling, chemical treatment, and other water purification methods are all effective, they can be time-consuming and labor-intensive. That's where portable water filters and purifiers come in. In this section, let's take a look at the different kinds and brands of portable water filters and purifiers available, and discuss some pros and cons of each. By no means is this a comprehensive list, but it will get you started on a great path.

Straw Filters

Straw filters are small, lightweight, and easy to use. They work by simply inserting the straw into a water source and sucking the water through. Many straw filters are designed to filter out bacteria and protozoa, but they may not remove viruses or other contaminants.

Popular brands include the LifeStraw, Sawyer Mini, and Aquamira Frontier.

Pros: Straw filters are very portable and easy to use, making them a great option for hikers and backpackers. They also require no batteries or other power sources, which can be a huge advantage in remote locations.

Cons: Straw filters may not remove all contaminants from water, and they can be difficult to use if the water source is shallow or difficult to access. They also need to be cleaned regularly to maintain their effectiveness.

Pump Filters

Pump filters are similar to straw filters, but they use a hand pump to force water through the filter. Many pump filters are capable of removing bacteria, protozoa, and viruses, as well as other contaminants like sediment and debris. Popular brands include the Katadyn Hiker Pro, MSR MiniWorks, and Platypus GravityWorks.

Pros: Pump filters are generally more effective than straw filters, and they are still relatively lightweight and portable. They also don't require any power source other than your own muscle power.

Cons: Pump filters can be more complex and difficult to use than straw filters, and they may require more maintenance. They can also be bulkier and heavier than straw filters, making them less suitable for ultralight backpacking.

Gravity Filters

Gravity filters work by allowing water to flow through a filter via gravity. They are often larger and more complex than straw or pump filters, and may be better suited for groups or families. Some gravity filters are capable of removing bacteria, protozoa, viruses, and even heavy metals and chemicals. Popular brands include the Platypus GravityWorks and the MSR AutoFlow.

Pros: Gravity filters are easy to use and can be very effective at removing contaminants from water. They are also relatively lightweight and portable, and may be a good option for groups or families.

Cons: Gravity filters can be bulkier and more complex than other types of filters, and may require more setup and maintenance. They may also be more expensive than other types of filters.

Chemical water purification tablets or drops

Purifying tablets can be an excellent choice for those who need a lightweight and portable water purification method for their outdoor adventures or emergency preparedness kits. The tablets can treat up to 30 gallons of water per package with treatment time taking as little as 15-30 minutes. Two of the most popular brands of chemical water purification products are Aquamira and Potable Aqua.

Pros: Chlorine dioxide tablets, which are highly effective against bacteria, viruses, and protozoa, and are easy to use - simply mix one tablet with water in a container, wait for the tablet to dissolve and then add it to the water that is about to be purified. One of the advantages of Aquamira tablets is that they don't leave any aftertaste in the treated water, which is a common complaint with other chemical treatments.

Cons: One important thing to note about chemical water purification is that it may not be effective against certain contaminants, such as heavy metals or chemicals. Additionally, some people may be sensitive to the chemicals used in the treatment process. One downside to iodine tablets is that they can leave a distinct aftertaste in the treated water, which can be unpleasant for some people. Iodine tablets are less effective against protozoa as well.

UV Purifiers

Discussed briefly earlier in the book, UV purifiers use ultraviolet light to kill bacteria, viruses, and other pathogens in water. They are often used in conjunction with other types of filters, as they are not effective at removing sediment or other debris. Popular brands include the SteriPen and the Grayl Ultralight.

Pros: UV purifiers are very effective at killing bacteria and viruses, and they are relatively lightweight and portable. They also don't require any chemicals or power sources other than batteries.

Cons: UV purifiers may not be effective at removing all types of contaminants from water, and they may require more maintenance than other types of filters. They may also be less effective in cloudy or turbid water.

By listing a few of the more popular portable water filter options on the market, along with my opinions of good and not so good points about each method, this should get you thinking and considering the best options for your situation. No matter which type of portable water filter or purifier that is chosen, it's important to carefully read the instructions and follow them closely. With a little bit of research and preparation, one can ensure that they always have access to clean, safe drinking water no matter where their outdoor adventures take them!

Chapter 4:

Water Safe Storage and

Transportation

"Water is life's matter and matrix, mother and medium. There is no life without water." —Albert Szent-Gyorgyi, M.D. Discoverer of Vitamin C

Access to safe and clean water is critical. However, ensuring that water remains safe to drink and use can be challenging, particularly when transporting and storing water. Improper storage and transportation can lead to contamination and pose a significant health risk. In this chapter, we will explore the best practices for storing and transporting water in emergency situations, including the importance of choosing the right containers, the proper methods for sanitizing water containers, and the best ways to store water for long-term use. By following these guidelines, one can ensure that their loved ones have access to safe and clean water when it is needed most.

Types of Water Containers

Choosing the right water container is a critical aspect of prepping. There are several types of water containers available for preppers, each with its unique advantages and disadvantages. In this section, we will explore the different types of water containers that preppers may use to be ready for a survival situation. As a disclaimer, this is not every type of water container available on the market, they are just some of my most trusted, most reliable options.

Plastic

Plastic water bottles are a popular choice for preppers due to their lightweight and easy-to-carry nature. They are also affordable and readily available. One of the main advantages of plastic water bottles is their portability, making them ideal for short-term use or when on the move. However, they are not suitable for long-term storage as plastic can degrade and leach chemicals into the water, compromising its quality. Additionally, plastic water bottles are not environmentally friendly as they contribute to waste and pollution.

Collapsible

Collapsible water containers are an excellent option for preppers who require a compact and lightweight storage solution. They can be easily stored in a bug-out bag, car, or other locations. Collapsible containers are usually made of durable materials such as BPA-free plastic or heavy-duty nylon, making them long-lasting and easy to clean. One of the disadvantages of collapsible containers is their smaller size, which may not be sufficient for long-term water storage needs.

Metal

Metal water containers are a durable and long-lasting option for preppers. They are usually made of stainless steel or aluminum and can withstand extreme temperatures and conditions. They are also resistant to corrosion and chemical leaching, making them an ideal choice for long-term water storage. However, metal containers can be heavy, making them less portable than other container types. They may also be prone to dents and scratches, which can compromise their integrity and make them difficult to clean.

Glass

Glass water containers are an eco-friendly and chemical-free option for preppers. They do not leach chemicals into the water, and their transparency makes it easy to monitor the water's quality. Glass containers are also easy to clean and can be reused multiple times. However, they are not as durable as other container types and can break easily, making them less suitable for outdoor activities or situations where they may be exposed to rough conditions.

Large Containers

Large water storage containers are ideal for preppers who require a significant supply of water for long-term storage. They can be made of various materials, including plastic, metal, and fiberglass. Large storage containers are usually equipped with features such as spigots, vent caps, and handles for easy access and portability. However, large containers can be heavy and bulky, making them difficult to transport, and they may require additional space for storage.

In conclusion, preppers have several options when it comes to water containers for survival situations. Each container type has its advantages and disadvantages, and preppers must choose the right container for their needs. It is also essential to ensure that the water containers are properly cleaned and maintained to prevent contamination and maintain water quality. By being prepared with the right water container, preppers can increase their chances of survival in emergency situations.

Sanitizing and Cleaning Water Containers

Now let's discuss one of the most important aspects of maintaining water containers - cleaning and sanitizing. I know what you're probably thinking: "cleaning and sanitizing? How boring!" But trust me, it's crucial for keeping water safe and healthy to drink. Think of it this way - if water containers are left dirty and bacteria-ridden, a person might as well just take a sip out of a swamp!

So, why is it so important to sanitize water containers? Well, let's start with the obvious. No one wants to drink water that's been contaminated with bacteria, mold, or other harmful substances. Not only can it make a person sick, but it can also affect the taste and smell of the water. And let's be real, nobody wants to drink water that smells like a musty old sock.

But it's not just about avoiding illness. Sanitizing water containers also helps to prevent the growth of algae and other microorganisms that can build up over time. This is especially important when storing water for an extended period of time, such as in an emergency situation. That water will be relied on to be as clean and safe as possible if the zombies come to visit, or more realistically, in a major catastrophe.

So, let's get down to the nitty-gritty. How does one actually clean and sanitize water containers? Well, it depends on the type of container being used. Let's start with the most common type - plastic containers.

Sanitizing Plastic Containers

First, empty out any water that's already in the container. Then, fill it up with a solution of 1 teaspoon of unscented bleach per gallon of water. Make sure the lid is securely fastened and then shake the container to distribute the solution throughout. Let it sit for at least 30 seconds, then pour out the solution and rinse the container thoroughly with clean water. Voila! That plastic container is now sanitized and ready to go. There are other methods here, but this one is my old standby that made the book.

Sanitizing Metal Containers

What about metal containers, you ask? The process is actually quite similar. Again, empty out any water that's already in the container. Then, fill it up with a solution of 1 teaspoon of unscented bleach per gallon of water. Make sure the lid is securely fastened and then gently swish the solution around to coat the entire interior of the container. Let it sit for at least 30 seconds, then pour out the solution and rinse the container thoroughly with clean water.

Sanitizing Glass Containers

Now, for those who prefer glass containers - don't worry, we haven't forgotten about you! Glass containers can be a bit more delicate than plastic or metal, so handle with a bit of care as to not damage them while cleaning. First, empty out any water that's already in the container. Then, fill it up with a solution of 1 teaspoon of unscented bleach per gallon of water. Gently swish the solution around to coat the entire interior of the container, being careful not to shake or bump the glass. Let it sit for at least 30 seconds, then pour out the solution and rinse the container thoroughly with clean water.

Mistakes to Avoid When Sanitizing

Now, before you all go off and start sanitizing every water container in sight, let's talk about a few common mistakes to avoid. First, make sure to use unscented bleach. Scented bleach can leave a residual odor that can be hard to get rid of. Second, don't forget to rinse the containers thoroughly with clean water after sanitizing. No one wants bleach or other cleaning solutions lingering in their water, gross! Finally, always make sure containers are completely dry before storing water in them. Moisture can lead to the growth of mold and other microorganisms.

So we made it through cleaning and sanitizing water containers correctly. This may not be the most exciting task, but it's a crucial step in ensuring that drinking water is safe and healthy. By following these simple steps and avoiding common mistakes, they will keep the sanitized water containers in tip-top shape and avoid any nasty surprises down the line.

Remember, when it comes to water storage and container maintenance, it's always better to be safe than sorry. Don't skimp on the cleaning and sanitizing - taste buds (and immune systems) everywhere are saying "THANK YOU!"

Storing Water for Emergency Situations

Today, when it comes to emergency preparedness, storing water is a crucial component. Water is an essential resource, and having a sufficient supply of it can mean the difference between survival and dehydration for you and your family. But where are the good and bad places to store water in your home?

Good Storage Areas

Good storage locations for water include cool, dark areas with a stable temperature. The ideal storage temperature for water is between 50 and 70 degrees Fahrenheit. Basements, closets, and other areas away from direct sunlight are good options. It's important to note that water stored in plastic containers should not be stored in direct sunlight or near heat sources as this can cause the plastic to degrade and contaminate the water.

Bad Storage Areas

On the other hand, bad storage locations for water include areas that are exposed to sunlight or extreme temperatures. Avoid storing water in garages, sheds, attics, or any other area that is not climate-controlled. Water stored in these areas is at risk of contamination and can be rendered undrinkable in a matter of days.

Now that we know where to store water, let's discuss why storing water is so important. In an emergency situation, access to clean drinking water may be limited, and the water supply could be compromised. Having a supply of stored water ensures that you and your loved ones have access to clean water for drinking, cooking, and hygiene purposes.

Storage Techniques

Preppers, who are known for their dedication to emergency preparedness, use various storage techniques to ensure a sufficient supply of water in a survival stockpile. These techniques range from simple to complex and depend on personal preference, available resources, and space limitations.

Some preppers use large, food-grade plastic barrels for long-term storage. These barrels are specifically designed for water storage and are capable of holding up to 55 gallons of water. Other preppers use smaller containers, such as 5-gallon jugs, which are easier to transport in case of an emergency. Some preppers even go as far as to install rainwater harvesting systems to collect and store rainwater for future use. Doing all 3 of these options is not a bad idea!

Mistakes to Avoid When Storing Water

Regardless of the storage technique, it's important to avoid common mistakes when storing water for an emergency. One common mistake is failing to rotate stored water regularly. Water that has been stored for a long period can become stagnant and develop an unpleasant taste. **It's recommended to rotate stored water every 6 months** to ensure that it remains fresh and palatable.

Another mistake is failing to properly sanitize water containers before storage. Any containers used for water storage should be thoroughly cleaned and sanitized to prevent the growth of harmful bacteria and microorganisms.

In summary, storing water for emergency situations is a crucial aspect of emergency preparedness. The key to effective water storage is to choose the right location and storage technique, and to avoid common mistakes such as failing to rotate stored water or failing to properly sanitize containers. With a little bit of preparation, it will ensure bountiful amounts of clean drinking water during any emergency for the whole family. That is peace of mind, so get to work!

Water Rotation and Maintenance

When it comes to storing water for emergencies, it's not just about finding the right location and container. You also need to keep an eye on the water itself and make sure it's properly maintained.

Rotation

One important aspect of water maintenance is rotation. Over time, stored water can become stagnant and develop an unpleasant taste. To prevent this, it's recommended to rotate your stored water every 6 months. This means using up the water that's been stored and replacing it with fresh water.

There are a few different ways to rotate that stored water. One way is by simply using it for everyday purposes, like watering plants or cleaning, and then refilling the containers with fresh water. Alternatively, pouring out the old water and using it for something else, like flushing toilets, before refilling the containers is an option.

It's important to make sure that someone is rotating this water on a regular basis. If forgotten about, there could be a nasty surprise waiting when an emergency situation arises. That is when the water is needed most, so be diligent, make a checklist if that works best, make this a habit to check on the water in the stockpile area, it will be worth it if say an EMP hits our country, or even if the power goes out from bad weather for an extended period. Remember shelter, food, protection are indeed important elements to figure out in a survival situation. However, most experts don't argue that water is the #1 crucial resource to obtain if facing an emergency event.

Upkeep

In addition to water rotation, general maintenance and upkeep of the water storage area and containers will be necessary. This includes regularly checking for leaks or damage to these containers, as well as cleaning and sanitizing them as needed. As I just mentioned, a checklist of tasks with these simple items on it will make this as easy as a walk in the park.

It's also important to keep your storage area clean and dry. If your storage area is damp or dirty, it can lead to the growth of mold and bacteria, which can contaminate that water supply.

By following these maintenance and rotation tips, it's fairly simple to ensure that the stored water is fresh, clean, and safe to drink in an emergency situation. And let's face it, in an emergency, the last thing someone wants is to be stuck drinking nasty, stagnant water. So, take care of that water supply, and it will take care of you when it's needed most!

Transporting Water - Methods and Safe Practices

When it comes to transporting water for emergency situations, it's important to have the right tools for the job. There are a variety of containers that can be used to transport water, each with their own pros and cons. Here's a list of some of the most common options:

Buckets

These are the simplest and most readily available containers for transporting water. They're easy to carry and can hold a decent amount of water. However, they're not the most practical for large-scale water transportation.

Pumps

If a person is in need of transporting a large volume of water, a pump can be a good option. They can move water quickly and efficiently, but they do require a power source and some setup time.

Hoses

Hoses can be used to transport water from one place to another. They're flexible and easy to maneuver, but they can be heavy and difficult to handle if they're very long.

Water Tanks

These are larger containers that can be used to transport a significant amount of water. They're typically mounted on a trailer or truck and are designed to be pulled behind a vehicle. While they're great for transporting water over long distances, they can be expensive and difficult to maneuver in tight spaces. Another thing to consider, if there is an extended catastrophe situation, these larger tanks draw attention. The less of a crowd the better if it's the only clean water in the neighborhood.

Barrels

These are sturdy containers that can be used to transport water in smaller quantities. They're often made of plastic or metal and can be easily transported in the back of a vehicle. However, they're not always the most efficient use of space and can be difficult to stack.

Drums

Similar to barrels, drums are another option for transporting water. They're typically larger than barrels and can hold a greater volume of water. However, they're heavier and more difficult to move around.

Tank Trucks

These are large vehicles designed specifically for transporting water. They can hold a massive amount of water and are great for long-distance transportation. However, they require a special license to operate and can be expensive to rent or purchase.

When choosing a container to transport water, it's important to consider 1) the specific needs for that water and 2) the distance needed to cover. Each container has its own strengths and weaknesses, so it's important to choose the one that's right for the situation at hand.

Mistakes to Avoid in Transporting Water

In addition to choosing the right container, there are certain mistakes that can be avoided to ensure the safe and efficient delivery of this vital resource. One of the biggest mistakes is not securing the container properly. If the container isn't properly secured, it could tip over or spill, causing damage to the vehicle or surrounding property.

Another mistake is overloading a container with water. It's important that the container is not carrying more weight than it can handle. Even along short distances, this can be a big problem. Overloading a water container can cause it to break or leak, which can be a disaster when trying to transport water in an emergency.

Inadequate packaging is one common mistake for transporting water. It's crucial to choose containers that are designed specifically for water transportation, such as sturdy plastic or stainless steel containers with secure lids. Using subpar packaging materials can lead to leaks, contamination, and loss of water during transit.

Another thing to consider during water transport is poor handling practices. Mishandling water containers during transportation can lead to damage and loss. It's important to handle the containers with care while loading, and while in motion. Avoid rough movements or impacts that can cause leaks or spills. Additionally, proper lifting techniques should be employed to prevent injuries to the individuals involved in the transport process.

Last but not least, ignoring regulatory requirements when transporting water can be a big problem. Transporting water may be subject to various regulations and permits, depending on the jurisdiction and the nature of the transport. It is important to be aware of and comply with all relevant laws and regulations governing the transportation of water. Failure to do so can result in legal consequences and potential disruptions to the water supply chain. Now in an evacuation, or disaster emergency these regulations may not be enforced, but they are listed here for your safety.

By choosing the right container and avoiding common mistakes, one can safely and effectively transport water in an emergency situation. Please remember, it's always better to be prepared ahead of time so you're not left scrambling in a crisis. Some situations are out of your control, such as natural disasters. Let's dive into our water for survival chapter of how you can be better prepared for when Mother Nature has other plans!

Chapter 5:

Water Emergency Situations and

YOU; Preparing for Catastrophes

"Water is the driving force of all nature." —Leonardo da Vinci

Water emergencies can arise at any time, and it is essential to be prepared for catastrophes. In natural disaster emergencies, such as droughts, floods, hurricanes, forest fires, blizzards, and tornadoes, it is crucial to have a plan in place for water preparation for your home and your loved ones. While some may think that preparing for water emergencies is only for the paranoid or the doomsday preppers, it is better to be safe than sorry. After all, as the famous saying goes, "it's better to have it and not need it, than to need it and not have it." The purpose of this chapter is to provide you with practical advice and real-life stories on how to prepare for and overcome contaminated water or water shortages during natural disasters. Some suggestions may be redundant, and some disasters may not apply to where you live. However, you never know where life may take you, so I will cover many situations that Mother Earth may throw at you. So, let's dive into this important topic, and remember, stay hydrated, my friends!

Drought

Droughts are a common occurrence in the United States, and they can strike almost anywhere. Droughts occur when there is a prolonged period of dry weather, leading to a shortage of water. They can be devastating, particularly for farmers and those living in rural areas. From the arid Southwest to the usually lush Southeast, no region is immune to the effects of drought. In fact, according to the National Centers for Environmental Information, between 1980 and 2020, the U.S. experienced 53 drought events that caused at least $1 billion in damages each. These events led to a total cost of over $289 billion! In this section, we'll explore how to prepare for drought and ensure that a typical U.S. family has enough water to last through the dry times if they follow these guidelines.

First, let's talk about where droughts typically occur in the United States. As mentioned, no region is entirely immune to drought, but some areas are more susceptible than others. The Southwest, for example, is a hotbed for drought, with Arizona, New Mexico, and Texas often experiencing prolonged dry periods. The Great Plains, including parts of Kansas, Nebraska, and Oklahoma, are also prone to drought due to their semi-arid climate. Meanwhile, California is another area that has experienced severe drought in recent years. The key is to know your region's drought patterns and to be prepared to adapt to a drier climate.

Now, let's talk numbers. As of January 2022, more than half of the United States is experiencing some level of drought, with areas like the Pacific Northwest and the upper Midwest are facing severe and exceptional drought. In 2020, more than 38 million people in the U.S. were affected by drought, with California, Arizona, and New Mexico facing some of the worst conditions. Drought can also have long-lasting effects, with the 2011-2017 California drought leading to a significant decline in the state's agriculture industry and costing the state over $2.7 billion in economic losses.

So, how best does one prepare for a drought? One of the most important things to do is to ensure that there is enough water to last through the dry times. This means taking a multi-faceted approach to water storage. First, evaluate local water sources. Is it from a well, or is it from municipal water? If it's water from a well, make sure that it is properly maintained and that there is a backup power source in case of a power outage. If the source is municipal water, consider investing in a water storage tank or barrels to store water in case of shortages.

Next, it's essential to ensure that the home is water-efficient. Fixing leaks, upgrading to low-flow toilets and showerheads, and only running full loads of laundry and dishes can all help to reduce the water usage. Additionally, consider installing a rainwater harvesting system, which can collect rainwater from the roof and store it for later use.

In 2014, California declared a drought emergency statewide, in the midst of one of the worst droughts in history. To overcome the water scarcity, residents took the following measures:

They limited their outdoor water use by reducing the frequency of watering their lawns and gardens.

They installed low-flow showerheads and faucets to reduce water usage.

They reused greywater from their washing machines and showers to irrigate their gardens.

Some benefits of these community measures are:

- Conserving water can help reduce water bills and save money.

- Installing low-flow showerheads and faucets can also save money on water bills.

- Reusing greywater can reduce the amount of wastewater sent to treatment plants.

When it comes to storing water for an emergency, there are a few common mistakes to avoid. First, make sure to have food-grade storage containers that are specifically designed for long-term water storage. Second, don't store water in direct sunlight or in a location where it is likely to freeze. Third, be sure to rotate the water supply regularly to ensure that it stays fresh and drinkable. Finally, don't forget to store water for those pets and livestock, if applicable. Some of this is redundant, but these are simple guidelines to ensure hard times are not tragic times.

Finally, it's important to have a plan for evacuation in case an evacuation becomes necessary. This may involve identifying safe routes out of the area and packing an emergency kit with essentials like food, water, and first aid supplies. Keep in mind that in a drought situation, local authorities may issue evacuation orders to protect public health and safety.

Flood

When it comes to natural disasters in the United States, floods can come on quickly and can cause devastating damage to homes and communities. Floods occur when water overflows from rivers, lakes, or oceans, causing damage to homes and properties. They can be caused by heavy rain, snowmelt, or storms. Knowing how to prepare for a flood can help minimize the impact on your life and property. In this section, we'll cover the basics of flood preparedness, including where floods typically occur in the U.S., statistics on floods in the United States, how to prepare your primary water source and home for a flood, and common mistakes to avoid when storing water for an emergency.

First, let's take a look at where floods typically occur in the U.S. Floods can happen anywhere, but they are most common in coastal areas, low-lying areas, and areas near rivers and streams. **In fact, according to the Federal Emergency Management Agency (FEMA), floods are the most common natural disaster in the United States, and they can happen in all 50 states.** Some states are more prone to flooding than others, however. For example, the state of Louisiana experiences an average of 118 floods per year, making it the most flood-prone state in the U.S. Here are some reasons to be prepared for floods:

- According to the National Oceanic and Atmospheric Administration, floods are the most common natural disaster in the United States.

- Flooding can cause significant damage to homes, resulting in costly repairs.

- Floods can lead to water contamination, which can cause waterborne diseases.

In 2017, Hurricane Harvey hit the Gulf Coast of Texas, causing massive flooding. The flooding caused water contamination, and residents were urged to boil their water before use. Many households were left without water, and some had to rely on bottled water for weeks. To overcome the water shortage, residents took the following measures:

- Residents collected rainwater for drinking and cooking.

- They filtered water using portable water filtration systems.

- People purchased bottled water from stores.

Some benefits of these community measures are:

- Collecting rainwater can be an inexpensive way to obtain water during a flood.

- Using portable water filtration systems can provide clean water during emergencies.

- Purchasing bottled water can provide a convenient source of clean drinking water.

Now that we know a bit about where floods occur in the U.S., let's take a look at some statistics on floods. According to FEMA, floods cause an average of $8.2 billion in damages in the U.S. each year. Additionally, floods are responsible for more deaths each year than any other type of natural disaster, with an average of 89 flood-related fatalities per year.

So, how do people prepare their water source and home for a flood? Like with droughts, the first step is to evaluate the water source. If the home or property is reliant on a well for its water supply, it's important to make sure that it is properly protected from contamination during a flood. Consider installing a backflow prevention valve and making sure that the well casing is above the highest flood level for your area.

If the property relies on a municipal water supply, check with the local water authority to find out if they have a plan in place for ensuring safe water during a flood. Typically homes in flooded areas need to boil their water before drinking it or use bottled water until the water supply has been deemed safe.

Next, it's important to prepare the home for a flood. If you live in a flood-prone area, consider elevating the house or building a flood wall or levee. Additionally, make sure that the sump pump is in good working order and that there is a battery-powered backup in case of a power outage.

Like ALL natural disaster situations, it's also important to have an emergency kit on hand that includes essentials like food, water, and first aid supplies. Additionally, make sure that there is a family evacuation plan in place if necessary, and that several family members are aware of the location of the nearest emergency shelter. One unique variable with a flood is the timing and how quickly things can escalate. Droughts will linger and there is time to consider options, where if a local levee breaks, a major river nearby overflows, or there is torrential rain overnight, the decision to evacuate or implement that emergency plan could be immediate.

In conclusion, floods are a common occurrence in the United States, and it's important to be prepared for these natural disasters. By evaluating the water source, preparing the home for a flood, and properly storing water for emergencies, a family can help to minimize the impact of a flood on their life. With a bit of preparation most families can be ready to weather the storm and come out on the other side unscathed.

Hurricane

Hurricanes are severe storms that can cause high winds, heavy rain, and flooding. These are annually, one of the most destructive natural disasters that can hit the U.S., particularly along the East Coast and the Gulf of Mexico. According to the National Oceanic and Atmospheric Administration (NOAA), the Atlantic hurricane season runs from June to November, with an average of 12 named storms per year. To prepare for a hurricane, it is important to secure the home by boarding up windows and doors, trimming trees and shrubs, and securing any loose outdoor items. No surprise, there should be at least 1 good disaster kit prepared with plenty of water, non-perishable food, a first-aid kit, flashlights, and batteries.

Hurricanes are one of the most destructive natural disasters and can cause widespread damage and disruption. According to the National Oceanic and Atmospheric Administration, hurricanes cause an average of $28 billion in damages each year in the United States. Access to clean water can become compromised during a hurricane due to power outages, flooding from ocean water, and other factors. Here are some tips on how to prepare your water source and emergency water reserves, as well as how to prepare your home for a hurricane.

Preparing Your Water Source and Emergency Water Reserves

Stock up on bottled water: In the days leading up to a hurricane, stock up on bottled water to ensure that you have enough to last for several days.

Fill containers with water: Fill clean containers with water for use in case of a power outage or flooding. Store these containers in a cool, dark place.

Consider a water filtration system: A water filtration system can be used to filter and purify water from natural sources such as rivers and streams.

Common Mistakes to Avoid in Preparing for a Hurricane

- Not preparing enough emergency water: During a hurricane, access to clean water can become compromised for several days or even weeks. It is important to stock up on enough emergency water to last for at least 72 hours.

- Not having a backup water source: In case of a power outage or other emergency, it is important to have a backup water source such as a well or rainwater collection system.

- Not testing emergency water reserves: Water stored for emergency use should be tested periodically to ensure that it is still safe to drink.

Preparing Your Home for a Hurricane

Secure windows and doors: To protect your home from damage during a hurricane, make sure that windows and doors are properly secured.

Have a backup power source: In case of a power outage, have a backup power source such as a generator or solar panels.

Trim trees and shrubs: Trim trees and shrubs around your home to prevent them from falling and causing damage during a hurricane.

In 2017, Hurricane Maria devastated Puerto Rico and left millions of residents without access to clean water. One family, the Fernandez family, had prepared for the storm by filling every container they could find with water and storing them in their garage. However, the storm was more severe than they had anticipated, and their home was flooded with contaminated water.

The Fernandez family quickly realized that their emergency water reserves were compromised and turned to a natural source: a nearby river. They used a portable water filtration system to purify the river water and were able to sustain themselves for several days until help arrived.

Despite the difficult circumstances, the Fernandez family was able to survive Hurricane Maria thanks to their preparedness and resourcefulness.

In conclusion, hurricanes can pose a serious threat to your water supply. To prepare for a hurricane, stock up on bottled water, fill containers with water, and consider a water filtration system. Avoid common mistakes such as not preparing enough emergency water or not having a backup water source. Additionally, prepare your home for a hurricane by securing windows and doors, having a backup power source, and trimming trees and shrubs. With the right preparation, you can weather any hurricane and ensure that you and your family have access to clean water during and after the storm.

Blizzard

Blizzards are severe winter storms that can bring heavy snow, high winds, and freezing temperatures. They can be dangerous, causing power outages and making it difficult to access clean water. Blizzards are more common in the northern parts of the country. According to the National Weather Service, the average snowfall in the U.S. is 28 inches per year, with some areas receiving up to 500 inches per year. During a blizzard, access to clean water can become compromised due to frozen pipes, power outages, and other factors. To prepare for a blizzard, make sure the home is well-insulated and the heating system is in good working order. There should also be plenty of blankets and warm clothing on hand, as well as a generator in case of a power outage.

Here are some tips on how to prepare your water source and emergency water reserves, as well as how to prepare your home for a blizzard.

Stock up on bottled water: In the days leading up to a blizzard, stock up on bottled water to ensure that you have enough to last for several days. Pro tip, do not store it outside!

Fill containers with water: Fill clean containers with water for use in case of a power outage or frozen pipes. Store these containers in a cool, dark place.

Melt snow for drinking water: In a pinch, snow can be melted and used for drinking water. However, be sure to melt snow over a heat source and filter the water before drinking.

Common Mistakes to Avoid When Blizzard is in the Forecast

Forgetting to insulate pipes: Frozen pipes can lead to a lack of running water during a blizzard. To prevent this, insulate pipes with foam or other insulation material.

Using unsafe water sources: During a blizzard, it may be tempting to melt snow or ice for drinking water. However, be sure to avoid using snow or ice that has been contaminated with chemicals or other pollutants.

Neglecting to test emergency water reserves: Water stored for emergency use should be tested periodically to ensure that it is still safe to drink.

Preparing Your Home for a Blizzard

Insulate windows and doors: To keep your home warm during a blizzard, make sure that windows and doors are properly insulated. If you live in Canada, or most of the midwestern United States, this is pretty standard. However, extra insulation is never a bad thing for noise, energy bills, and obviously warmth in your home.

Have a backup heating source: If your home relies on electricity for heating, have a backup heating source such as a generator or wood-burning stove. I have detailed lists of options in my book New Prepper's Survival Bible.

Keep emergency supplies on hand: In case of a power outage or other emergency, have a stockpile of emergency supplies such as food, water, and blankets. A stove for cooking,(and heating) along with fuel to run it up is a nice thing to store in your survival gear.

In 2013, a blizzard hit South Dakota, leaving thousands of residents without power or running water. One family, the Henderson's, had prepared for the storm by stockpiling bottled water and filling their bathtub with water for emergency use.

As the storm raged on, the Henderson's ran out of bottled water and their bathtub water began to run low. However, they had a plan in place: they melted snow for drinking water using a camping stove and coffee filters to filter out impurities.

Despite the harsh conditions, the Henderson's were able to survive the blizzard thanks to their preparedness and resourcefulness.

Blizzards can pose a serious threat to your water supply. To prepare for a blizzard, stock up on bottled water, fill containers with water, and be prepared to melt snow for drinking water if absolutely necessary. Avoid common mistakes such as neglecting to insulate pipes or using unsafe water sources. Additionally, prepare your home for a blizzard by insulating windows and doors, having a backup heating source, and keeping emergency supplies on hand. With the right preparation, you can weather any blizzard and ensure that you and your family have access to clean water during and after the storm.

Tornado

Tornadoes are violent forces of nature that can strike suddenly and leave behind significant damage to properties & livestock. Tornadoes are a common occurrence in the central and southern regions of the U.S., often referred to as "Tornado Alley." According to the National Oceanic and Atmospheric Administration (NOAA), there are an average of 1,200 tornadoes per year in the U.S. In the aftermath of a tornado, access to clean water can be compromised due to damage to water infrastructure or contamination of water sources. To prepare for a tornado, all family members should identify a safe place in the home, such as a basement or interior room, and make sure all family members know where to go in case of an emergency.

Here are some tips on how to prepare your water source and emergency water reserves, as well as how to prepare your home for a tornado.

Stock up on bottled water: In the days leading up to a tornado, stock up on bottled water to ensure that you have enough to last for several days.

Fill containers with water: Fill clean containers with water for use in case of a power outage or damage to water infrastructure. Store these containers in a cool, dark place.

Consider a water filtration system: A water filtration system can be used to filter and purify water from natural sources such as rivers and streams.

Collect rainwater for non-potable uses: often rain follows a tornado, rain from the heavens could be in abundance, if there is no structural damage, plus it is an inexpensive way to collect water for important uses.

Preparing Your Home for a Tornado

Identify a safe room: Identify a safe room in your home where you and your family can take shelter during a tornado.

Secure windows and doors: To protect your home from damage during a tornado, make sure that windows and doors are properly secured.

Have a backup power source: In case of a power outage, have a backup power source such as a generator or solar panels.

In 2011, an EF5 tornado struck Joplin, Missouri, and left behind significant damage. One resident, Mike Stoll, had prepared for the storm by filling several 5-gallon buckets with water and storing them in his basement. However, the storm was more severe than he had anticipated, and his home was destroyed.

Despite the destruction, Mike was able to access one of his water storage containers and use it to sustain himself until help arrived. He also used a water filtration system to purify water from a nearby river.

The aftermath of the Joplin tornado left behind a contaminated water supply, but Mike's preparedness and resourcefulness allowed him to access clean water and survive in the days after the storm.

Tornadoes can have a significant impact on your water supply. To prepare for a tornado, stock up on bottled water, fill containers with water, and consider a water filtration system. If you are seeing a theme here with prepping your water source for natural disasters it's intentional. Avoid common mistakes such as not preparing enough emergency water or not having a backup water source. Additionally, prepare your home for a tornado by identifying a safe room, securing windows and doors, and having a backup power source. With the right preparation, you can survive a tornado and ensure that you and your family have access to clean water during and after the storm.

Wildfires

Wildfires are a major concern in many parts of the U.S., particularly in the western states. According to the National Interagency Fire Center, there were over 58,000 wildfires in the U.S. in 2020, burning over 10 million acres. To prepare for a wildfire, make sure the home is not located in a high-risk area and that the property is clear of any debris or flammable materials. The disaster kit I keep suggesting ... Yes, have one handy for the family that can be easy to bug out with if the fire gets too close.

Wildfires can also pose a significant threat to your water supply. During a wildfire, water infrastructure can be damaged, and water sources can become contaminated, leaving you with limited access to clean water. Here are some tips on how to prepare your water source and emergency water reserves, as well as how to prepare your home for a wildfire.

Fill containers with water: Fill clean containers with water for use in case of a power outage or damage to water infrastructure. Store these containers in a cool, dark place. Many families in high risk wildfire areas will keep fire pump backpacks on hand. These are collapsible bags that you can wear & spray areas to keep wet or extinguish if they are on fire.

Consider a water filtration system: A water filtration system like a Berkey, can be used to filter and purify water from natural sources such as rivers and streams. Keep one of these in your home and you will not be disappointed.

Keep your property clear of flammable materials: Clearing dry brush, dead leaves, and other flammable materials from around your property can help prevent wildfires from reaching your home and contaminating your water sources.

Preparing Your Home for a Wildfire

Create a defensible space: Clearing dry brush and other flammable materials from around your home can create a defensible space that can help protect your home from wildfires.

Install ember-resistant vents: Ember-resistant vents can help prevent embers from entering your home and starting a fire.

Close all windows and doors: During a wildfire, close all windows and doors to prevent embers from entering your home and contaminating your water sources.

In 2018, the Camp Fire swept through the town of Paradise, California, leaving behind significant damage. One resident, Dave Garrett, had prepared for the fire by filling up his bathtub with water and shutting off the main water supply to his home to prevent contamination from the fire.

However, the fire was more severe than he had anticipated, and his home was destroyed. Despite this, Dave was able to access the water in his bathtub and use it to sustain himself until help arrived.

The aftermath of the Camp Fire left behind a contaminated water supply, but Dave's preparedness and resourcefulness allowed him to access clean water and survive in the days after the fire.

Wildfires can have a significant impact on your water supply. With the right preparation, you can survive a wildfire and ensure that you and your family have access to clean water during and after the fire.

Earthquake

Earthquakes can happen anywhere in the U.S., but are more common in the western states along the Pacific Coast. According to the U.S. Geological Survey, there are an average of 20,000 earthquakes per year in the U.S., with most being too small to be felt. To prepare for an earthquake, make sure the home is structurally sound, and secure any heavy furniture or objects to prevent them from falling over. An earthquake can strike without warning, leaving everyone in the area without access to clean and safe drinking water. When an earthquake strikes, it's important to turn off the home's water supply to prevent contamination. After the earthquake, check the water supply for damage or leaks before using it for drinking or cooking. If the water supply has been compromised, use that stored water supply we've been discussing this entire book, until the water is deemed safe by local authorities.

Like many of the already listed natural disasters in this chapter, earthquakes too can disrupt your families water supply and cause damage to infrastructure, leaving you without access to clean water. To prepare for an earthquake and ensure that you have access to clean water, here are some tips on how to prepare your water source and emergency water reserves, as well as how to prepare your home.

Store water in a safe location: Store clean water in containers in a safe and accessible location. It is important to have enough water for at least three days.

Install a water filtration system: Install a water filtration system that can filter and purify water from natural sources such as rivers and streams.

Have backup water sources: Consider having backup water sources such as a well or rainwater collection system in case of damage to water infrastructure.

Preparing Your Home for an Earthquake

Secure water heaters and tanks: Secure water heaters and tanks to prevent them from falling and causing damage to water infrastructure.

Install shut-off valves: Install shut-off valves that can be used to turn off water in case of damage to water infrastructure.

Inspect water lines and pipes: Inspect water lines and pipes for damage and have them repaired or replaced if necessary.

In 2010, a 7.0 magnitude earthquake struck Haiti, causing significant damage to infrastructure and leaving many without access to clean water. One resident, Nadine Pierre, had prepared for the earthquake by storing water in plastic bottles and filling up her bathtub with water before the earthquake struck.

After the earthquake, Nadine was without access to clean water for several days. She was forced to ration the water that she had stored and boil water from a nearby river to make it safe to drink. She also shared her water with neighbors who did not have access to clean water.

Despite the challenges, Nadine was able to survive and access clean water by being prepared and resourceful.

Earthquakes are scary and can cause severe long-term damage. With taking these preventative steps and combined with some common sense (and a little luck) the items discussed above can increase you and your families odds of getting through an earthquake with clean and fresh water afterwards.

In addition to preparing your home and family for natural disasters, it is important to have a plan for your #1 resource, **water!** Natural disasters can strike at any time and can leave households without access to clean water for days, even weeks on-end. The recommended amount of water to have on hand is 1 gallon per person per day for at least 3 days, I'd recommend 14 days if space allows for it. Having a plan for water preparation can help households overcome water shortages and water contamination during natural disasters. By collecting rainwater, purchasing bottled water, using water filtration systems, and boiling water before use, you can ensure your household will have a source of clean water when Mother Nature decides to wreak havoc in your neck of the woods. Preparing for a natural disaster can be a daunting task,but remember to create an emergency kit, stay informed, be prepared, and above all, stay safe. Additionally, evacuation to safer areas may be necessary in some cases. Being prepared and having a disaster-ready plan in place can make a significant difference in ensuring the safety and well-being of loved ones during natural disasters. Please don't forget to keep a sense of humor even in the face of disaster. After all, laughter is the best medicine, and sometimes it's the only thing that can get you through tough times.

Man-made Disasters

When preparing for natural disasters, it's important to remember that man-made disasters can also occur. Man-made disasters refer to catastrophic events that are caused by human activities, negligence, or error. These disasters can have a significant impact on the water supply in an emergency. Here are some examples:

Chemical spill

Chemical spills can occur due to accidents in transportation or industrial facilities. These spills can contaminate water sources, making it unfit for human consumption. In an emergency, your water supply may be cut off or limited due to contamination, and you may need to find an alternative source of water.

Oil Spills

Oil spills can occur due to accidents in transportation or oil rigs. These spills can also contaminate water sources, making it unfit for human consumption. In an emergency, your water supply may be cut off or limited due to contamination, and you may need to find an alternative source of water.

Nuclear Accidents

Nuclear accidents can occur due to failures in nuclear power plants or other nuclear facilities. These accidents can release radioactive material into the environment, including water sources. In an emergency, your water supply may be cut off or limited due to contamination, and you may need to find an alternative source of water.

Infrastructure Failures

Infrastructure failures can occur due to aging or lack of maintenance. Examples include water main breaks or dam failures. In an emergency, your water supply may be cut off or limited due to infrastructure failure, and you may need to find an alternative source of water.

Terrorism

Acts of terrorism, such as intentional contamination of water sources, can have a significant impact on the water supply in an emergency. In such cases, it is important to follow guidance from authorities on finding alternative sources of water or treating water before consumption.

In all of these scenarios, it is important to have a plan in place for accessing alternative sources of water, such as bottled water or water purification methods, in case your regular water supply is compromised. In these types of disaster situations, access to clean water can be a matter of life or death. Here are some reasons to prepare your water source in advance, as well as some common mistakes to avoid.

Reasons to Prepare Your Water Source in Advance

Limited access to clean water: In a disaster situation, the municipal water supply may become contaminated or disrupted. By preparing your water source in advance, you can ensure that you have access to clean water when you need it.

Increased demand for bottled water: In the aftermath of a disaster, bottled water can quickly become scarce. By preparing your water source in advance, you can avoid the rush and ensure that you have enough water for your family.

Protection from contamination: In a man-made disaster, chemical spills or other contaminants may enter the water supply. By preparing your water source in advance, you can protect your family from exposure to these harmful substances.

In 2014, the city of Toledo, Ohio was hit with a man-made disaster when toxic algae blooms in Lake Erie contaminated the city's water supply. The algae blooms were caused by agricultural runoff, and the toxins in the water could cause nausea, vomiting, and liver damage.

The city issued a do-not-drink order, leaving 400,000 residents without access to clean water. In response, residents rushed to stores to buy bottled water, quickly emptying store shelves.

However, one local resident, David Lauer, had prepared his water source in advance. Lauer had a rain barrel system installed at his home, which collected rainwater from his roof and stored it in a 250-gallon tank.

When the do-not-drink order was issued, Lauer and his family were able to use the rainwater from their tank for drinking, cooking, and cleaning. They even shared their water with neighbors who had not prepared in advance.

In an interview with CNN, Lauer said, "We feel very grateful that we had this system in place. It's a lot of peace of mind."

The Toledo water crisis serves as a reminder of the importance of preparing your water source in advance. By taking the time to store and treat your water, you can ensure that you and your family have access to clean water in even the most challenging situations.

In conclusion, it's important to remember that man-made disasters can also impact your water source. By preparing your water source in advance, you can ensure that you have access to clean water when you need it. Avoid common mistakes such as failing to store enough water or using improper storage containers, and rotate your stored water every six months. With the right preparation, you can overcome any disaster and protect your family's health and safety.

Evacuation Planning

When a natural disaster strikes, having a solid family evacuation plan in place can make all the difference. Here are some important considerations to keep in mind when preparing a family evacuation plan:

Identify potential evacuation routes: Research potential evacuation routes in the immediate area, including alternate routes in case those primary routes are blocked. Consider having multiple evacuation plans for different types of natural disasters, such as hurricanes, floods, or wildfires. If Florida is home, no need to have a plan for blizzard evacuations, please use common sense people.

Choose a meeting place: Decide on a meeting place where the whole family can reunite in case anyone gets separated during the evacuation. Make sure everyone knows the location and how to get there.

Pack essential items: Prepare a "go bag" with essential items such as food, water, medication, first aid supplies, and important documents. Each family member should have their own go bag, and it should be stored in an easily accessible location. There are tons of internet resources just on this topic. I will not go into detail here but one of my other book's The New Prepper's Survival Bible, has a whole chapter dedicated to just this topic.

Bring water for the journey: Water is one of the most important items to account for during an evacuation. Pack enough water to last each family member for at least three days (7 days if possible), and consider investing in portable water filters or purification tablets to ensure access to clean water during the evacuation.

Prepare for pets: Don't forget to include those 4 legged friends in the evacuation plan! Make sure the pets have enough food, water, and supplies, and consider pre-arranging a place to stay with friends or family that can accommodate those furry friends as well.

Stay informed: Keep up-to-date with the latest information from local authorities, and be prepared to adjust the evacuation plan as needed. Consider signing up for emergency alerts on your phone, and keep a battery-powered radio on hand for updates in case of power outages.

Practice the plan: Finally, practice the catered evacuation plan with the whole family to ensure everyone knows what to do in case of a natural disaster. Go over the plan regularly, and make adjustments as needed to ensure everyone is as prepared as possible. There may be some resistance at first, or this may seem awkward, but have fun with it and keep it light.

In summary, having a solid family evacuation plan in place can help keep your loved ones safe during a natural disaster. By identifying potential evacuation routes, choosing a meeting place, packing essential items, bringing water with you, preparing for pets, staying informed, and practicing the plan, everyone can be ready to evacuate at a moment's notice in the event of a natural disaster.

Chapter 6:

Water-borne Diseases

"Nothing is softer or more flexible than water, yet nothing can resist it." —Lao Tzu

Water-borne diseases are a silent killer that lurks in our water sources and threatens our health. These diseases can be caused by a variety of agents, including viruses, bacteria, parasites, and chemicals that are present in our water supply. While water is essential to our survival, it can also be a source of danger if not treated properly. In this chapter, we will explore the world of water-borne diseases, starting with a clear definition of what they are and the different types that exist. We will then delve into the causes of these diseases, providing examples of how they can contaminate our water sources. We will also discuss the mechanisms of transmission, highlighting the various ways in which these diseases can be spread. Additionally, we will examine the symptoms and effects of water-borne diseases, as well as the preventive measures that can be taken to keep ourselves and our loved ones safe. By the end of this chapter, you will have a better understanding of water-borne diseases and be equipped with the knowledge to protect yourself and your community from these dangerous illnesses.

As a prepper, it's essential to recognize the importance of water for survival. However, it's not enough to just have access to water. One must also ensure that the water they are consuming is free of contaminants, including water-borne diseases. A water-borne disease is an illness caused by drinking or being exposed to water that contains harmful bacteria, viruses, or parasites. Water-borne diseases can cause severe illness, hospitalization, and even death in some cases.

In North America, water-borne diseases are more common than one might think. In fact, according to the Centers for Disease Control and Prevention (CDC), approximately 7.15 million people in the United States are affected by water-borne diseases every year. That's an incredibly high number coming from one of the most developed nations in the world, and it highlights the importance of being vigilant about the quality of your drinking water.

One particularly alarming example of the dangers of water-borne diseases occurred in 1993 in Milwaukee, Wisconsin. In that year, over 400,000 people were infected with the Cryptosporidium parasite, which was present in the city's drinking water supply. The outbreak resulted in 69 deaths and over 4,000 hospitalizations. The incident remains one of the largest water-borne disease outbreaks in U.S. history and serves as a stark reminder of the importance of taking water quality seriously.

This event demonstrated that no matter how advanced a nation's infrastructure is, the threat of water-borne diseases is always present. As a prepper, it's essential to prepare for situations like this and ensure that you have access to clean, safe water. This means having a reliable water source that is free from contaminants and taking measures to treat your water if necessary.

In summary, water-borne diseases are a real and serious threat, and they can have devastating consequences for those who consume contaminated water. The example of the 1993 Cryptosporidium outbreak in Milwaukee serves as a reminder that water-borne diseases can occur in even the most developed nations. Therefore, it's essential for preppers to take steps to ensure that their water is clean and safe for consumption in any situation. By doing so, preppers can protect themselves and their families from the dangers of water-borne diseases and increase their chances of survival in an emergency situation.

Causes of Water-borne Diseases

Water-borne diseases can be caused by a variety of contaminants that exist in our water sources. These contaminants can range from microorganisms like bacteria and viruses to chemicals and heavy metals. It's important to be aware of the different causes of water-borne diseases and take steps to mitigate them to ensure the safety of your water supply.

One of the most common causes of water-borne diseases is bacterial contamination. According to the World Health Organization (WHO), bacterial infections are responsible for 80% of all water-borne disease cases. Some of the most common bacterial contaminants found in water sources include E. coli, Salmonella, and Shigella.

Another cause of water-borne diseases is viral contamination. In North America, the norovirus is one of the leading causes of viral water-borne diseases. The norovirus can cause severe gastrointestinal symptoms like vomiting and diarrhea, and it's highly contagious, making it a serious threat to public health.

Parasitic infections are also a significant cause of water-borne diseases. Cryptosporidium and Giardia are two common parasitic infections found in water sources that can cause severe gastrointestinal symptoms.

Chemical contamination is another cause of water-borne diseases, and it can be caused by natural or man-made sources. For example, arsenic contamination is a natural occurrence that can cause severe health effects when consumed in drinking water. Man-made chemicals like pesticides and industrial chemicals can also contaminate water sources and cause health problems.

One example of the dangers of chemical contamination occurred in Flint, Michigan in 2014. The city's drinking water supply was contaminated with lead due to aging water infrastructure and inadequate treatment. The incident resulted in widespread health effects, particularly in children, and highlighted the need for proper water management and infrastructure investment.

In conclusion, water-borne diseases can be caused by a variety of contaminants, including bacteria, viruses, parasites, and chemicals. As a citizen, it's essential to be aware of these causes and take steps to mitigate them to ensure the safety of the water supply. The example of the Flint water crisis serves as a stark reminder of the dangers of chemical contamination and the importance of proper water management and infrastructure. This is an ongoing struggle today as of this writing in 2023 in Flint. By understanding the causes of water-borne diseases and taking appropriate measures, most people have the ability to protect themselves and their families from the dangers of contaminated water.

Types of Infections

There are numerous examples of water-borne diseases that can affect humans. Some of the most common water-borne diseases include:

- **Cholera**: A bacterial infection caused by the bacterium Vibrio cholerae, which can cause severe diarrhea and dehydration.

- **Typhoid fever**: A bacterial infection caused by the bacterium Salmonella typhi, which can cause fever, abdominal pain, and severe diarrhea.

- **Hepatitis A**: A viral infection caused by the hepatitis A virus, which can cause liver inflammation and jaundice.

- **Cryptosporidiosis**: A parasitic infection caused by the parasite Cryptosporidium, which can cause severe diarrhea.

- **Giardiasis**: A parasitic infection caused by the parasite Giardia, which can cause severe diarrhea and abdominal cramps.

- **Legionnaires' disease**: A bacterial infection caused by the bacterium Legionella pneumophila, which can cause severe pneumonia and respiratory problems.

- **Norovirus**: A viral infection that can cause severe gastroenteritis, including diarrhea, vomiting, and stomach cramps.

- **E. coli infection**: A bacterial infection caused by the bacterium Escherichia coli, which can cause severe diarrhea, vomiting, and abdominal cramps.

- **Dysentery**: An infection caused by several different bacteria, viruses, and parasites, which can cause severe diarrhea and abdominal pain.

It's important to note that water-borne diseases can have serious health effects, particularly for vulnerable populations like children, the elderly, and those with weakened immune systems. Therefore, taking steps to prevent water-borne diseases, such as using safe drinking water sources, treating water appropriately, and maintaining good hygiene practices, is essential for protecting public health.

Transmission

One of the biggest risks associated with consuming contaminated water is the potential for water-borne diseases to spread. There are several mechanisms of water-borne disease transmission, and understanding these can be critical in preparing for survival situations.

One common mechanism of water-borne transmission is through the ingestion of water that has been contaminated with fecal matter. This can occur when sewage or animal waste contaminates water sources, or when human waste is not properly disposed of. In fact, according to the Centers for Disease Control and Prevention (CDC), the most common causes of water-borne illness in the United States are associated with fecal contamination of water supplies.

Another mechanism of water-borne transmission is through the ingestion of water that has been contaminated with pathogenic organisms, such as bacteria or viruses. These organisms can cause a range of illnesses, from mild gastroenteritis to more severe infections like cholera and typhoid fever. In addition to ingestion, some water-borne diseases can also be transmitted through skin contact, inhalation of contaminated water droplets, or through contact with contaminated surfaces or objects.

According to the World Health Organization (WHO), water-borne diseases are responsible for an estimated 3.4 million deaths each year, with the majority of these occurring in low-income countries. However, water-borne diseases can also pose a significant risk in North

America. For example, in 1993, a large outbreak of cryptosporidiosis occurred in Las Vegas, Nevada, resulting in over 400,000 cases of illness and several deaths. The outbreak was traced to contamination of the city's water supply with the parasite Cryptosporidium, which had been introduced through a contaminated water source.

Another notable example occurred in Walkerton, Ontario, Canada, in 2000. Following heavy rainfall, contamination of the town's water supply occurred due to agricultural runoff containing E. coli bacteria. Over 2,000 cases of illness were reported, with seven fatalities. The incident led to a public inquiry and significant changes in the way water is treated and monitored in Canada.

To prepare for survival situations, it's important to consider the mechanisms of water-borne transmission and take steps to mitigate these risks. One way to do this is by investing in water treatment options, such as portable water filters or chemical treatment kits, which can help to remove or inactivate harmful pathogens. In addition, it's important to avoid consuming water from questionable sources, such as streams or standing bodies of water, which may be more likely to contain harmful contaminants.

Hygiene, Food, and Contaminated Water

In addition to contaminated water sources, poor hygiene practices and unsafe food preparation practices can also contribute to mechanisms of water-borne disease transmission.

Good hygiene practices, such as washing hands regularly with soap and water, particularly before preparing food or eating, and avoiding contact with potentially contaminated surfaces or objects will lower the risk. One common example of this is when individuals fail to wash their hands properly after using the bathroom. If these individuals then handle food or touch surfaces that others may come into contact with, they can potentially spread harmful pathogens that can cause water-borne illness.

Other hygiene practices, such as the sharing of utensils, cups, or towels, can also contribute to the spread of water-borne disease. In survival situations, it may be more difficult to maintain proper hygiene practices, especially if there are limited resources or facilities available. This highlights the importance of being prepared and having appropriate supplies on hand to help maintain hygiene and prevent the spread of illness.

Another example is when food is prepared in an unsanitary manner, such as when raw meat or other contaminated ingredients are not properly cleaned or stored. This can result in harmful bacteria or viruses contaminating food, which can then cause illness when consumed. In addition, safe food storage and preparation practices should be followed, such as cooking meat to appropriate temperatures and avoiding consumption of raw or undercooked food.

Overall, understanding the various mechanisms of water-borne disease transmission is critical in preparing for survival situations. To prevent the spread of water-borne disease through poor hygiene practices and unsafe food preparation, it is important to follow good hygiene practices, including washing hands regularly, cleaning food, and food preparation surfaces, and avoiding cross-contamination. Understanding the mechanisms of water-borne transmission and taking steps to mitigate these risks can help to protect against water-borne illness and promote public health.

Symptoms

Water-borne diseases can have a wide range of symptoms and effects, depending on the specific pathogen involved and the severity of the illness. In the United States, some of the most common water-borne diseases include giardiasis, cryptosporidiosis, and norovirus, among others.

Symptoms of water-borne illness can include diarrhea, nausea, vomiting, abdominal pain, fever, and dehydration. In severe cases, some individuals may experience life-threatening complications such as kidney failure, meningitis, or even death.

Let's explore the critical importance of handling water-borne diseases in emergency situations, and how individuals can prepare and respond if faced with a crisis where access to clean water is limited and possibly consumed.

Jenna was an experienced hiker who loved to explore the great outdoors. She was well prepared for her latest adventure, packing a backpack filled with all the essentials she needed to survive in the wilderness. But despite her preparations, she soon found herself in a dire situation.

Jenna had run out of clean water and had no way of getting more. She was forced to drink from a nearby stream, which she knew was not safe to drink. However, she was so thirsty that she drank from it anyway, hoping for the best.

Soon after, Jenna began to feel sick. She had a fever, stomach cramps, and diarrhea. She knew she had contracted a waterborne illness from the contaminated water she had drunk. She was miles away from civilization and knew that she had to rely on herself to survive.

Jenna remembered the advice she had read about boiling water to make it safe to drink. She gathered some wood, started a fire, and boiled some water from the stream. She let it cool, and then drank it. Slowly but surely, Jenna began to feel better. She continued to boil water and drink it until she was able to find a clean water source.

Jenna's experience taught her the importance of boiling water in survival situations. Without access to clean water, she could have become seriously ill or even died. Boiling water is just one of several simple and effective ways to make water safe for consumption, and it can save lives in emergency situations. Overall, Jenna's story highlights the importance of access to clean water and the need for preparation and knowledge in survival situations. By being aware of potential water sources and knowing how to purify them, we can ensure our own safety and survival when venturing into the great outdoors.

While many individuals may recover from water-borne illness within a few days to a week, there can be long-term health effects for some. These can include chronic digestive problems, kidney damage, and even neurological issues such as cognitive impairment or depression. This highlights the importance of taking steps to prevent water-borne illness, as the consequences can be far-reaching and severe.

Several risk factors can increase an individual's likelihood of developing severe illness from water-borne diseases. These can include:

1. **Age**: Infants, young children, and the elderly are often at higher risk for developing severe illness from water-borne diseases due to weaker immune systems and other factors.

2. **Immunocompromised status**: Individuals with weakened immune systems, such as those with HIV/AIDS, cancer, or who are undergoing chemotherapy, are at higher risk for developing severe illness from water-borne diseases.

3. **Underlying health conditions**: Individuals with underlying health conditions such as liver disease, diabetes, or other chronic illnesses may also be at increased risk for severe illness from water-borne diseases.

4. **Exposure to contaminated water sources**: Individuals who live in areas with poor water quality or who travel to areas with higher rates of water-borne disease may be at increased risk for developing illness.

5. **Poor hygiene practices**: As discussed earlier, poor hygiene practices can increase the risk of transmitting water-borne pathogens, which can in turn increase the risk of severe illness.

In order to protect themselves and their loved ones from water-borne illness, individuals can take several steps to reduce their risk. These can include:

Boiling or treating water: Boiling water can be an effective way to kill harmful pathogens and make water safe to drink. Other methods such as using water purification tablets or filters can also be effective.

Maintaining good hygiene practices: This includes washing hands regularly, avoiding sharing cups or utensils, and practicing safe food preparation practices.

Storing water properly: Water should be stored in clean, airtight containers to prevent contamination.

Monitoring water quality: Individuals who live in areas with poor water quality can monitor local advisories and take appropriate precautions.

Seeking medical attention if necessary: If symptoms of water-borne illness develop, it is important to seek medical attention to receive appropriate treatment and prevent complications.

By understanding the common symptoms and effects of water-borne disease, as well as the risk factors for severe illness, individuals can take proactive steps to protect themselves and their families. In survival situations, access to safe and clean water can be a critical factor in maintaining health and well-being. By being prepared and knowledgeable about water-borne disease prevention, individuals can better ensure their own survival and promote the health of their communities.

In conclusion, water-borne diseases remain a serious threat to public health in North America and around the world. From the various types of diseases, to the causes and mechanisms of transmission, it is clear that proper hygiene and safe water management practices are essential for preventing these illnesses. The symptoms and effects of water-borne diseases can range from mild to severe, and long-term health effects can have a significant impact on individuals and communities. Education and awareness are also crucial in the fight against water-borne diseases. By educating individuals and communities about the risks associated with these illnesses and promoting safe water management and hygiene practices, we can reduce the incidence and spread of water-borne diseases. Governments, organizations, and individuals must work together to improve water management and sanitation practices. By making the necessary investments in infrastructure and education, we can create a future where everyone has access to safe and clean water. It is our responsibility to protect ourselves and our communities from the threats posed by water-borne diseases. Let us all take action and work towards a future where water-borne diseases are a thing of the past.

Chapter 7:

Water Rationing, Public Education, and the Future of Water Conservation

"When the well's dry, we know the worth of water." –Benjamin Franklin

Water is the essential resource for human survival, and its conservation and efficient use are critical for both personal and environmental health. Despite being one of the most abundant substances on Earth, fresh, clean water is scarce in many parts of the world. As the global population continues to grow, so does the demand for water, making it a precious and valuable resource. Per the U.N. World Water Development report in 2023 26% of the world's population still does not have access to safe drinking water and 46% lack access to basic sanitation. That global population number is 7.9 billion and rising daily. Staggering, because in other words 1 in 4 people on our planet do not have daily clean water!

In emergency situations, water scarcity can become a life-threatening issue. As discussed earlier, natural disasters, such as floods, droughts, and hurricanes, can severely impact the availability and quality of water, leaving communities without access to clean and safe water. In these situations, water rationing is often necessary to ensure everyone has access to the basic levels of water to survive.

The chapter will delve into the importance of water conservation and the role of water rationing in emergency situations. It will also explore the significance of public education in promoting the need for clean water everyday, including when we may be face to face with a survival situation. In addition, the chapter will discuss the different techniques and technologies used for water conservation, such as rainwater harvesting, wastewater treatment, and water-efficient appliances.

Overall, the chapter will emphasize the importance of water conservation, rationing, and public education in promoting water sustainability and ensuring access to clean water in emergency situations. The chapter aims to raise awareness about the importance of water and its responsible use, highlighting the need for individuals, communities, and governments to work together to achieve water security and sustainability.

Water conservation

Water conservation is critical for preserving and protecting our freshwater resources. Conserving water is not only beneficial for the environment, but it can also help save money on water bills, reduce energy consumption, and ensure water availability during times of drought or emergency. In this chapter, we will discuss some facts on water conservation, tips on how best to conserve water in your daily life, and how to best conserve water for emergency situations. We will also discuss some things to avoid in proper water conservation.

Facts on Water Conservation

- Approximately 70% of the earth's surface is covered in water, but only 2.5% of it is freshwater.

- The average person in the US uses around 80-100 gallons of water per day.

- A leaky faucet can waste up to 20 gallons of water per day.

- The use of low-flow showerheads, faucets, and toilets can save up to 50% of the water used in a home.

- Approximately 75% of the water used in a home is used in the bathroom.

- Agriculture accounts for 70% of the world's freshwater consumption.

- Around 30% of the world's population lacks access to safe drinking water.

Tips on Water Conservation in Daily Life

- **Fix leaks**: Fixing leaks in faucets and toilets can save a significant amount of water. Even a minor drip can waste gallons of water per day, which can add up over weeks or months to your water bill as well.

- **Use low-flow fixtures**: Switching to low-flow fixtures such as showerheads, faucets, and toilets can reduce water usage significantly.

- **Take shorter showers**: Reducing the time spent in the shower can save a considerable amount of water.

- **Turn off the tap**: Turn off the tap when brushing teeth, washing dishes, or shaving. This will absolutely conserve water, and is a good habit.

- **Use a broom**: Use a broom instead of a hose to clean driveways and sidewalks.

- **Water plants efficiently**: Water plants early in the morning or late in the evening when temperatures are cooler to reduce evaporation.

- **Collect rainwater**: As discussed in multiple chapters already, collecting rainwater in a barrel or bucket can provide a source of water for plants and gardens.

Tips on Water Conservation for Emergency Situations

- **Store water**: In an emergency, it is crucial to have a supply of water on hand. Store at least one gallon of water per person per day for at least three days.

- **Use water-efficient appliances**: Using water-efficient appliances such as low-flow toilets and showerheads can help conserve water during an emergency.

- **Treat water**: If no clean water is available, it is essential to treat the available water. Boiling water, using a water filter or purification tablets, or using bleach can make water safe to drink.

- **Reuse water**: In an emergency, it is crucial to conserve as much water as possible. Reusing water can help conserve water. For example, the water used for washing dishes can be used for flushing toilets. If you own a RV, or camp, this should be easy to follow.

Things to Avoid in Proper Water Conservation

- **Letting the water run unnecessarily**: Letting the water run while brushing teeth or shaving can waste a considerable amount of water.

- **Overwatering plants**: Overwatering plants can lead to water wastage and promote the growth of mold and other fungi.

- **Using hoses for cleaning**: Using a hose for cleaning instead of a broom can lead to water wastage.

- **Using a dishwasher or washing machine with a half load**: Running a dishwasher or washing machine with a half load can waste water and energy.

In conclusion, water conservation is critical for ensuring water security and sustainability. Conserving water in daily life and during emergency situations can help protect freshwater resources, save money, and reduce energy consumption. By following the tips mentioned above and avoiding wasteful practices, we can all play a part in conserving water for future generations.

Water Rationing

Water rationing is a practice implemented by many communities and organizations to conserve water during times of drought or other water shortage situations. In the United States, water rationing guidelines are set by the state and local governments, as well as various water management organizations. These guidelines are critical to ensure that water resources are used efficiently and sustainably, especially during emergencies and natural disasters.

According to the U.S. Environmental Protection Agency (EPA), the average American uses about 80-100 gallons of water per day. This includes water used for drinking, washing, and irrigation, among other purposes. However, water scarcity and drought conditions are becoming more prevalent across the United States, making it necessary to ration and conserve water resources.

One of the most notable organizations for water conservation in the US is the Alliance for Water Efficiency (AWE). AWE is a non-profit organization that focuses on promoting sustainable and efficient water use in North America. They provide resources and information for individuals, businesses, and organizations to help them conserve water and reduce water waste.

Another notable organization is the American Water Works Association (AWWA), which is the largest nonprofit, scientific, and educational association dedicated to managing and treating water in the world. AWWA provides guidelines, tools, and resources to help utilities and communities manage water resources effectively and sustainably.

In times of drought or emergency, states and local governments may implement water rationing guidelines to ensure that water is distributed efficiently and fairly. These guidelines may include restrictions on water usage, and enforcing reduced hours for commercial water users. Understanding these guidelines is critical for individuals and communities to conserve water resources and prevent water shortages. Below is a compiled list from several of these sources regarding typical community guidelines for water rationing that a person can adopt into their daily life.

- **Prioritize essential needs**: Ensure that essential needs such as drinking water, cooking, hygiene, and sanitation are met first.

- **Assess daily water usage**: Keep track of daily water usage and identify areas where water can be saved.

- **Limit outdoor water use**: Avoid watering lawns and landscaping as well as washing the family vehicles during times of drought or water shortage.

- **Wash clothes and dishes efficiently**: Use full loads and the appropriate water-saving settings on washing machines and dishwashers.

- **Reuse gray water**: Reuse water from sinks, showers, and washing machines for tasks like watering plants.

- **Use drought-tolerant plants**: Consider planting drought-tolerant vegetation in landscaping.

- **Limit non-essential activities**: Avoid activities that consume large amounts of water, such as filling pools or hot tubs.

- **Use water-efficient appliances**: Using water-efficient appliances such as low-flow toilets and showerheads can help conserve water. When buying new appliances, look for those with the WaterSense label, which indicates that they meet water efficiency standards.

- **Don't run half-loads in the dishwasher or washing machine**: Running a dishwasher or washing machine with a half load can waste water and energy. Wait until you have a full load before running these appliances.

- **Avoid using the toilet as a trash can**: Flushing trash down the toilet can waste a lot of water. Use a trash can instead.

- **Public education**: Raise awareness of water conservation through public education and communication campaigns.

Water rationing guidelines are essential for ensuring sustainable water use in the US, especially during times of drought and emergencies. With organizations such as AWE and AWWA, individuals and communities can access information and resources to conserve water and reduce water waste. By following these tips, and adopting water conservation practices, we can protect our freshwater resources for future generations.

Water Education

Public education on the importance of clean water rationing in survival situations is crucial. It can help people understand the risks of water contamination and the need for proper water treatment and conservation practices. Educating the public about water conservation can lead to behavioral changes that support the efficient use of water resources, resulting in the sustainable use of freshwater. By integrating water conservation into the curriculum, educational institutions can equip students with the knowledge and skills necessary to make informed decisions about water usage. Through educational initiatives, individuals learn about the importance of water as a finite resource, the impacts of excessive consumption, and the methods to conserve and protect water sources. Public education also extends beyond the classroom, involving outreach programs, community events, and digital platforms to engage the wider public in the conversation.

By incorporating age-appropriate lessons, projects, and interactive activities, schools can instill a sense of environmental responsibility and empower students to become advocates for water conservation. The curriculum can cover topics such as the water cycle, water scarcity, sustainable water management, and the role of individuals in conserving water. By fostering a culture of conservation early on, students are more likely to carry these values into adulthood, thereby creating a sustainable impact on water usage.

Through comprehensive public education and communication campaigns, we can raise awareness, foster responsible attitudes, and inspire sustainable water usage, safeguarding this precious resource for future generations.

Conclusion

Final Word

Water is the most critical resource for survival in any situation. From the depths of the wilderness to the heart of the city, we all rely on water to sustain us. However, despite the fact that water is so essential to our lives, it is all too easy to take it for granted. It is only in situations of scarcity or emergency that we truly appreciate the value of water. In a disaster situation, access to clean drinking water is often the difference between life and death. Water is required not just to hydrate ourselves, but also for cooking, cleaning, growing, and sanitation.

I have outlined the importance of water and how to secure a clean and reliable water source, as well as how to purify and store water for emergencies. On this journey, I have shared a few wild stories of survival related to water, and have passed along many facts on water for survival for you to have forever in this guide. Also, various lists for tips and tricks have been discovered that are fairly easy to implement into your life today! Finally, I have discussed the importance of water rationing and the role that it plays in ensuring that essential needs are met, and how education is crucial.

However, all of this information is useless unless it is put into action. We call on all preppers to take this information and put it into practice. Take the time to research and understand the water sources in the area, and implement the best methods for securing and purifying water. Share this information with friends and family, and encourage them to take water survival seriously as well.

But perhaps the most important lesson we can learn from the importance of water in survival situations is the need to respect and value this precious resource. We must not take water for granted, assuming that it will always be there when we need it. Instead, we must take responsibility for our water usage, conserve water where we can, and work to protect our water resources for future generations. In the end, the importance of water for survival is not just a matter of life and death. It is a reminder of our interconnectedness with the natural world, and our responsibility to care for the planet that sustains us.

In these uncertain times, it is more important than ever to be prepared for emergencies. By making water survival a priority, we can ensure that we are ready for anything that comes our way. Remember, the key to survival is preparation, and the more handbooks like this one in your home library, the better odds of success for surviving, and even thriving, in a worst-case scenario event! So, let's take action today and ensure that we have a secure and reliable source of water for tomorrow. Let us remember the lessons of water and strive to build a more sustainable and resilient world. For when we honor the importance of water, we honor the very essence of life itself!

Sources List

Chapter 1

https://www.offgridweb.com/survival/alone-in-the-sahara-the-survival-story-of-mauro-prosperi/

https://www.nationalacademies.org/news/2004/02/report-sets-dietary-intake-levels-for-water-salt-and-potassium-to-maintain-health-and-reduce-chronic-disease-risk

Chapter 2

https://www.wikihow.com/Build-a-Rainwater-Collection-System

https://www.medicalnewstoday.com/articles/what-percentage-of-the-human-body-is-water

Chapter 3

https://www.backdoorsurvival.com/how-important-is-reverse-osmosis-for-drinking-water-filtration/

https://www.science.gov/topicpages/w/water+filtration+ion-exchange

https://drinking-water.extension.org/drinking-water-treatment-ozone/

Chapter 5

https://www.ncei.noaa.gov/access/billions/

Chapter 6

https://www.cdc.gov/healthywater/surveillance/burden/index.html

https://www.mlive.com/news/flint/2023/01/bottled-water-dries-up-in-flint-as-water-crisis-fallout-continues-in-new-year.html

Chapter 7

https://www.epa.gov/watersense/water-conservation-plan-guidelines

https://savewatersantafe.com/water-conservation-rules-and-regulations/

https://www.awwa.org/Policy-Advocacy/AWWA-Policy-Statements/Water-Use-Efficiency

https://www.npr.org/2023/03/22/1165248040/1-in-4-people-in-world-lack-clean-drinking-water-u-n-says

www.ingramcontent.com/pod-product-compliance
Lightning Source LLC
Chambersburg PA
CBHW022101020426
42335CB00012B/785